The Hardstyle Kettlebell Challenge

A Fundamental Guide to Training for Strength and Power

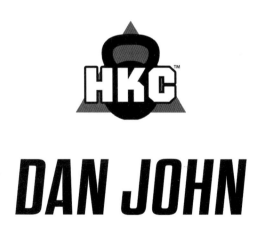

DAN JOHN

Advance Praise for

The Hardstyle Kettlebell Challenge

"Dan John is one of the premier strength coaches on the planet. I was thrilled to see him focus a book on the fundamental aspects of kettlebell training, the HKC. The kettlebell swing, goblet squat, and Turkish get-up represent movements that have been a foundation of my own strength programming for both my patients in the clinic, and fitness clients in the gym. I have seen profound changes in health and performance using Hardstyle kettlebell methods, from the fire fighter recovering from a low back injury, to training partners at my Brazilian Jiu Jitsu academy.

Dan breaks down the core Hardstyle kettlebell movements like no one else. I thought I had a firm grasp of the technique, programming, and application of the swing, get-up, and goblet squat until I read this amazing book. He truly goes a mile deep on the subject with no fluff, and filled in the missing pieces for me that I didn't even know I had. This is an absolute must read for any coach or trainer looking to incorporate kettlebells into their clients' training. The HKC is also a great starting point for the average person wanting to start strength training but is lost in the internet sea of (mis)information overload.

I give Dan John's ***The Hardstyle Kettlebell Challenge*** my highest recommendation, absolutely essential reading for the coach or trainee."
—**Chris Hardy**, D.O. MPH CSCS, Physician and Strength Coach, Author of Strong Medicine

---

"If you're serious about strength training, you study Dan John. If you're serious about kettlebells, you study Hardstyle. ***The Hardstyle Kettlebell Challenge*** gives you both. What more could you want?"
—**Pat Flynn**, author of *Paleo Workouts For Dummies*

"Coaches with Dan John's breadth of experience and knowledge are few and far between. Even rarer is one who can articulate their ideas so clearly, and in such an entertaining manner.

Dan has an uncanny ability to draw parallels between seemingly unrelated topics and put difficult concepts into words we can all understand.

Mr. John's incredible combination of world-class teaching skills and phenomenal writing talent make *The Hardstyle Kettlebell Challenge* an essential read for any fitness trainer or serious student of strength.

My primary training modality isn't even kettlebells—it's calisthenics—but this book still gave me ideas and insights I could immediately put to use."
—**Al Kavadlo**, PCC Lead Instructor, co-author of *Get Strong*

"Dan John has created, with The Hardstyle Kettlebell Challenge, the definitive book on not only kettlebell training but common sense training with any tool. Dan has taken the tools of the HKC (the Swing, Goblet Squat and Get Up) and (finally) given them their due! While many will discount these humble tools, they are missing the powerful benefits that deeply exploring them will being the athlete. From execution to programming, Dan has covered all the bases with this book. If you are an RKC, and HKC, or even a kettlebell neophyte you will benefit from the information in this book... and if you know someone who is using kettlebells then do them a HUGE favor and get them a copy of this book. They will thank you..."
—**Michael A. Krivka**, Sr.; Master RKC, Training Director - CrossFit Koncepts and Martial Arts Koncepts

---

"This book is an example of why Dan John has become one of the great trainers of our time. It is full of immediately applicable kettlebell drills for any fitness level. His mastery of the system is expressed with a simplistic calm. Like a patient mentor, he takes time for the details to get things right. Hardstyle Kettlebell Training will earn you a lasting strength, resilient joints and a hard physique. This book offers many programming options to keep the progress coming."
—**Robert A. Miller**, Senior RKC Instructor

"Much like the HKC itself, Dan John's HKC book drills down to the absolute essentials of kettlebell strength and conditioning. Ultra-practical, the HKC book includes all the necessities, how to use them, plus how to create programs for nearly any fitness level or athletic need.

While some may think that the three exercises of the HKC, the swing, get-up, and goblet squat can't possibly be enough, after 7 years as an RKC, and 6 as an RKC-II, Dan John's HKC book has inspired me to simplify my training, and that of my clients—with great results. The "basics" are so important to Hardstyle kettlebell training, and this book doesn't just make that case, it shows you exactly how to implement these crucial basics. I would recommend this book for kettlebell instructors and enthusiasts at all levels."
—**Adrienne Harvey**, Senior PCC, RKC-II, CK-FMS

"In everything I have ever read from Dan John, from his books, his blogs, or even a Facebook post, Dan has a unique ability to simplify training concepts, tactical approaches, and exercise procedures. This new book follows the same simplistic formula. Dan John is taking the HKC, which in itself is a simple introduction into learning the kettlebell and has dissected the 3 exercises that can be applied to a high-powered athlete, senior adult, young person just starting out, or to the everyday exercise freak that walks into your gym. I love this book. It's easy to follow, and Dan John tells great stories to make his points. I can't wait to pass along this knowledge."
—**Beth Andrews**, Senior RKC

"I love everything about *The Hardstyle Kettlebell Challenge*. In addition to the best writing I've ever seen on the swing, the goblet squat and the get-up, Dan John treats his readers to multiple discussions of larger concepts, time tested wisdom, and realistic coaching tips. One of my favorite sections is the brilliant passage on programming, where Mr. John evokes Woody Allen, stating that 90% of success in fitness and performance is "simply showing up."

Dan John has the gift (or is it just experience?) of taking extremely complex concepts and making them simple. So much of this book left me nodding my head as I read the words. The information contained within these pages is indispensable, yet easily approachable. Truly, the author's humor, wisdom and personal anecdotes make *The Hardstyle Kettlebell Challenge* a fantastic read!"
—**Danny Kavadlo**, PCC Master instructor, author of *Strength Rules*, co-author of *Get Strong*

"From the very beginning, I was blown away by the information in The Hardstyle Kettlebell Challenge. Dan John has a gift. He writes for the general public and his books and articles are always enjoyable.

I have been certified as an RKC since 2009 and have been a Senior RKC for a couple of years. I've been to many RKC certifications as both a participant and a team leader. Like Dan mentions in this book, I always learn something new. I learn new drills to bring to my clients to help them get better. I learn again how important my own practice is to make me a better trainer.

In his new book, Dan goes way beyond anything I've learned so far. This book is packed with tips, cues and exercises that I have never used with myself or my clients. Programming using just the HKC knowledge in combination with the many other exercises and drills that Dan teaches in this book is enough to give a new Kettlebell instructor an arsenal of tools to get their clients to their goals.

I am excited to take the knowledge to my clients. The book not only will help me to become a better Kettlebell instructor, but it will also help me improve as a coach to my Special Olympic powerlifters.

The Hardstyle Kettlebell Challenge is not only great for Kettlebell instructors, it's a comprehensive guide for coaching other sports, working with regular clients and doing your own training."

—**Laurel Blackburn**, Senior RKC and owner of Tallahassee Kettlebells, Boot Camp Fitness and Training and The Tallahassee Strength Club

The Hardstyle Kettlebell Challenge

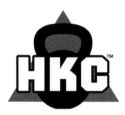

© Copyright 2017, Dan John
A Dragon Door Publications, Inc. production
All rights under International and Pan-American Copyright conventions.
Published in the United States by: Dragon Door Publications, Inc.
5 East County Rd B, #3 • Little Canada, MN 55117
Tel: (651) 487-2180 • Fax: (651) 487-3954
Credit card orders: 1-800-899-5111 • Email: support@dragondoor.com • Website: www.dragondoor.com

ISBN-10: 1-942812-12-4   ISBN-13: 978-1-942812-12-8
This edition first published in November 2017
Printed in China

No part of this book may be reproduced in any form or by any means without the prior written consent of the Publisher, excepting brief quotes used in reviews.

BOOK DESIGN: Derek Brigham • www.dbrigham.com • bigd@dbrigham.com

PHOTOGRAPHY: Mary Carol Fitzgerald • marycarolfitzgerald.com

DISCLAIMER: The authors and publisher of this material are not responsible in any manner whatsoever for any injury that may occur through following the instructions contained in this material. The activities, physical and otherwise, described herein for informational purposes only, may be too strenuous or dangerous for some people and the reader(s) should consult a physician before engaging in them. The content of this book is for informational and educational purposes only and should not be considered medical advice, diagnosis, or treatment. Readers should not disregard, or delay in obtaining, medical advice for any medical condition they may have, and should seek the assistance of their health care professionals for any such conditions because of information contained within this publication.

— Table of Contents —

Foreword by Mark Fisher

What is the HKC? 1

Why the HKC? 9

Programming the HKC 77

General Principles for the "Rest of Us"
Lessons from Elite Athletics 109

About the Author 137

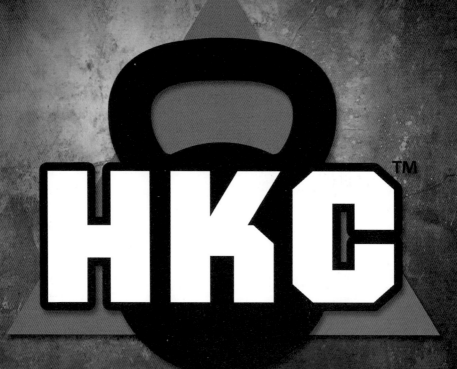

Foreword

By Mark Fisher

Like many in the fitness industry, I consider Dan John our resident philosopher-poet-king.

After many years of following his work from afar, I feel very lucky to now count Dan a personal friend and mentor. And it all began at a Hardstyle Kettlebell Certification (HKC) in Clayton, MO...

I still remember flying from NYC all by my lonesome because I was committed to doing whatever it took to experience the HKC with Dan. The original date had been pushed back because Dan's hip surgery had become time sensitive. And the reason I remember this is because Dan, who barely knew me at the time, *personally* called me to break the news of the postponement.

In the fall of 2011, the time had finally arrived, and off to Clayton, MO I went to learn from one of my heroes. It was a mild but cloudy day. I got into my rental car, found Stefanie Shelton's Studio RKC, and quietly entered.

Lo and behold, the event was intimate enough for us all to spend time together connecting on breaks and talking shop about our shared passion. If you've been in the field, you know the kind of conversation I'm talking about. Trading book recommendations, brainstorming on challenging client situations, sharing effective cues, etc.

And it was here I felt safe enough to take a risk and opened up about my personal style of coaching and teaching...

Now for those not familiar with Mark Fisher Fitness, you should know that our culture is, shall we say, "eccentric." We call our clients Ninjas, our mascot is the unicorn, and instead of calling our homes "gyms," we prefer to call them Enchanted Ninja Clubhouses of Glory and Dreams.

At the time I met Dan, MFF-the-organization was simply a twinkle in my eye. So it was with no small amount of trepidation that I began to share my approach with *THE* Dan John and the other attendees. By this time, I'd begun to codify how I teach movement technique and my training philosophy with many colorful images and metaphors. Some of it too colorful to reprint in polite company!

And in perhaps the ultimate example of Dan's kindness and vision... he immediately "got it."

He could see that the insane metaphors and over-the-top imagery were actually carefully considered teaching tools. My hope was to share the best practices of Dan and my other mentors in a way that was fun, accessible, and memorable. Since I was successful developing a niche working with NYC's Broadway community and other assorted "non-gym folk," I knew my approach was landing with my target audience.

But I can't quite put into words what it meant to receive Dan's vigorous and enthusiastic validation that day in Clayton.

In the years since, Mark Fisher Fitness has grown from a single weird personal trainer into a robust community of Ninja and coaches with two locations in Manhattan.

In one of the most serendipitous strokes of MFF's good luck, Dan's brother-in-law, the inimitable Geoff Hemingway, walked into our facility shortly after we opened. At the time, he was a Broadway actor looking to train amongst his Broadway brethren at MFF. Several years later, Geoff is now one of our superstar trainers and a pillar of our community. He's known as "Mr. Wonderful" around these parts, and if you ever have the good fortune to meet Geoff, you'll instantly see it's a fitting moniker. So it's not hyperbole to say Dan's officially "in the family."

Like any fitness facility, we're of course not perfect. We genuinely strive to be an industry leader in making the experience fun and inclusive while providing a best-in-class training experience for the general population. On the one hand, we look to create a space where people are seen as completely perfect, exactly as they are. On the other hand, we want to inspire our Ninjas to nudge 1% closer to their "ideal self." As you may imagine, this balance is hard. Some days we do better than others, but all in all, we're all pretty proud of what we've created.

And as we've pursued this North Star, we've been incredibly fortunate to have a secret weapon along the way; Dan John.

Since that fateful day in Clayton, I've continued to study Dan's work just as diligently as ever. I read his books and articles, I watch him speak live at conferences, and I stream his videos. And now we have a whole team of trainers to absorb, discuss, and apply Dan's wisdom.

Beyond our careful study of his work, Dan has graciously functioned as "adjunct faculty" to MFF. He's done in-services for our team and Ninjas, co-taught training sessions, and contributed in ways large and small to our never-ending quest for progress.

I'd be hard pressed to boil down Dan's influence on MFF. But I think it's much more foundational than specific exercises, coaching cues, or progressions.

In my humble opinion, here's what's so important about Dan's work in general, and the HKC in specific:

Principles.

Dan understands principles. And this is a rare gift.

Scientists tell us that organisms trend to increasing levels of complexity. You see this in almost all fields of human achievement, and fitness is no exception. It is easy, as Dan told me that cloudy day in Clayton, MO, to be "sitting on a whale, fishing for minnows." To get lost in the minutiae. To become entranced by fancy anatomical terms and (overly) sophisticated systems.

Yet somehow Dan's work gets *simpler* and *clearer* over time. His principles become more distilled as he relentlessly pursues savage excellence at the basics.

And while there is most certainly a time and place for mastery of details, they have no context without a set of underlying principles.

And Dan's work is all about reminding us of the principles. Or in the words of Johann Wolfgang von Goethe, "the things that matter most must never be at the mercy of the things which matter least."

Thankfully, by choosing this book, you can strap yourself in for a heaping dose of reasonableness. The HKC is more than a "workout." It's a philosophical foundation that will make you better as a coach. Dare I say it, this approach will make you a better *whatever it is you're trying to become in your life.*

These pages are an expression of one of Dan's core principles: mastery of the basics leads to mastery.

The Hardstyle Kettlebell Challenge represents an incredible platform to set you up for success as a fitness professional, strength coach, or kettlebell enthusiast. You have made a great investment in purchasing this book, and my hope is you savor the wisdom in its pages and apply its principles straightaway.

Before you head off into the book proper and begin feasting on Dan's wisdom and insight, let me offer one final thought.

Another overriding theme of Dan's work is an understanding that we're all part of a grand lineage of physical culturists. We're all standing on the shoulders of giants, and the only thing we can be sure of is that everything old will be new again eventually.

I for one feel grateful to have Dan's formidable shoulders to stand on.

And now you too, dear reader, are part of this noble lineage.

I hope that your deep dive into the Hardstyle Kettlebell Challenge under Dan's tutelage brings you some of the magic it's brought to my life and to an entire army of Ninjas here in NYC.

Mark Fisher

What is the HKC?

The longer I am involved in the Dragon Door kettlebell community, the more I take away from the simple concept of "Hardstyle." Understanding Hardstyle was a bit of a journey for me.

From my education background, I know that "both/and" answers tend to be a bit more elegant and encompassing. But, in coaching we face "either/or" answers all the time—either we win or we are out of the playoffs. So, when it came to something like Hardstyle, I really wanted someone to just tell me, "This is it!"

At first, complex things are rarely that simple. But later, complex things are that simple!

Yes, Hardstyle is from the Martial Arts tradition of "Force meets Force."

And it blends the softer movements of the restorative movements of Tai Chi.

And it teaches us to understand tension and relaxation.

And, yes Hardstyle includes the Yin-Yang relationship between the ballistic movements and the grinding movements. (Ballistics are the snatch and swing; Examples of grinds are squats and presses.)

Learning to turn on extreme tension has value for planks and perhaps the powerlifts (squat, bench press and deadlifts). Becoming as loose as possible has great application in restorative work, flexibility, and mobility training.

But, the ability to snap into high tension from relaxation is the master quality of sports.

It's called many things: from stretch-reflex to "bow and arrow," but the ability to apply the right amount of tension and relaxation at the appropriate moments is the secret to elite performance.

I can explain this by simply snapping my fingers. With the right tension in my thumb and middle finger along with the appropriate release, I will make a nice little popping sound. If I totally relax, no noise comes from my palm. If I totally tense, nothing happens!

The Hardstyle Kettlebell Three—the swing, goblet squat and get-up—are the gateway to understanding this crucial concept in fitness and performance. Athletes who snap, win. Those of us who can still pop up, leap into the fray, and bound into the office do better in life, living and everything else.

If you are interested in living longer, knowing how to roll on the ground will save your life in some situations, while leaping away will be the survival key to other life or death moments. Sometimes, you might just need to duck down—in that moment you will be glad to have been doing squats in your training.

The HKC Three introduce us to the concepts of elite performance. Frankly, I think anybody who trains on a regular basis is pretty elite since most people don't do any exercise at all. So, if you are training, then you are elite! Sometimes juggling life and training is a feat worthy of a superhero.

While we have named this method Hardstyle, it also goes by other names. When I was first introduced to throwing, the concept of "Bow and Arrow" was the standard method of teaching the finish of the throw. For the discus, shot and javelin we were told to drive our hips and chest into the direction of the throw and then let the "bowstring"—the energy in the body—snap the arrow/implement off into the sector. If one had the patience to let the implement stay back until releasing the bowstring, then amazing things happened.

Forty plus years later, I still can't think of a better way to teach the throws. We have tried to "science it up" with phrases like "pre-stretch" and "lateral chains" among many others, but the image of the bow and arrow is practically perfect "in every way" (with a nod to Mary Poppins). The body releases the elastic energy built up during the momentum-gathering phase (turn, glide or run up) and transfers it to the throw.

When done correctly, throwing, kicking and punching almost seem effortless when compared to the results. It's like simply pulling then releasing a rubber band that snaps over several rows of school desks to hit your best friend's earlobe.

Teaching the feeling of melding tension and relaxation is the cornerstone of the Hardstyle kettlebell method. And, we have a secret to teaching it. And like most secrets in life such as "buy low, sell high," it is sadly obvious. It is a painful truth much like Criss Jami noted, "Never hide things from hardcore thinkers. They get more aggravated, more provoked by confusion than the most painful truths."

The secret is no secret. It is a painful truth.

With the kettlebell swing, the hinge is the "bow" and the finish is the "arrow". When I first started doing swings correctly—please make sure you understand that, I said "correctly"—I immediately noticed an improvement in my throws. My first article about kettlebells noted this "What the Heck Effect" as I added nearly seventy feet to my javelin throw.

In all honesty, I wasn't much of a javelin thrower, but the difference astounded me! Suddenly, instead of trying to "huck and chuck" the javelin, my inner Spartan was snapping it off.

That's the power of the kettlebell swing. Performed correctly, the swing mimics the key to athletic success. However, there is another layer to sports performance. It took me years to understand it, but the journey was worthwhile.

Doctor Stu McGill is a legendary back researcher and all around good guy. He understands athletics and athletes because he studies them—he is also unique because he listens to them. He never rushes to judgment on corrections, regressions and progressions. Instead, he takes his time to make sure the answer actually fits the question.

I have sat in his lectures on many occasions, but only recently grasped his insight of the "hammer and stone". When he studies athletes, especially after they begin to struggle, he has observed that they often maintain high levels of power, hypertrophy and strength. Yet, their performance still begins to lag.

It took me a while to appreciate his insights about performance. The "hammer" is the explosive drive off of the ground, the hit, or the punch. The "stone" is the athlete's body. As we age, we might not lose our hammer, but we lose our stone!

Now, some caveats—keeping the stone is not necessarily maintaining six-pack abs, lean body mass and toned, tight and tanned buttocks. Instead it is the ability to hold together "in one piece", as I say in one of my three key principles of training:

1. The body is one piece.

2. There are three kinds of strength training: putting weights overhead, picking them up off the ground, and/or carrying them for time or distance.

3. All training is complementary.

Stone training is the connecting point of three concepts crucial to performance. Performance is the moment they call your name, turn on the spotlight, and the maestro taps the baton. You might be the best of the best in your gym or garage, but performance happens on the stage. A good set of stones are crucial in more ways than one when it comes to performance!

I've identified three interrelated types of stone training:

Anaconda Strength

I love using goofy names to explain concepts to athletes. Anaconda strength is the internal pressure we must exert to hold ourselves steady against the forces of the environment or an implement. A highland game athlete tossing a caber is fighting forces in every direction, yet maintaining his or her body as "one piece." Anaconda strength is the body squeezing and the inner tube of the body pushing back to keep integrity.

Armor Building

This is the kind of training that fighters, football teams and rugby athletes already understand. Armor building is the development of callouses or body armor to withstand the contact and collisions with other people and the environment.

Arrow

This is the concept of learning how to turn yourself into stone. In football, this the contact in tackling and blocking; in throwing, it is the block to put the energy into the implement.

Football, rugby, and collision occupations need all three kinds of stone training. Olympic hammer throwers need anaconda strength, while javelin throwers (with a much lighter tool) simply need to learn to zap themselves into an arrow.

The easiest way to explore stone training is to first acknowledge that you need it. The most basic way to realize this to work on the movements I often call the "Moving Planks." The goblet squat and the get-up are moving planks—as is the top of the kettlebell swing. The HKC really is the answer to all questions.

There are a few small variations of the goblet squat that can help teach inner pressure (the anaconda strength).

Goblet squat curls

At the bottom of the goblet squat, lock your elbows into your knees and perform some curls. Note how the body needs to counter this movement. By the way, this is the movement that made me name my arms "armacondas."

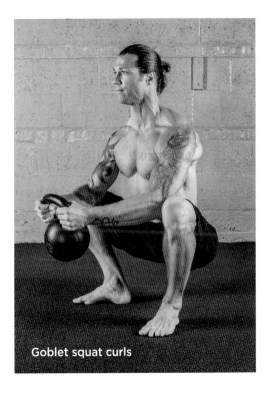

Goblet squat curls

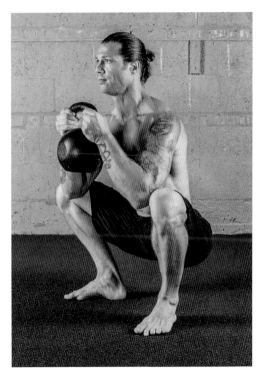

Goblet squat heartbeats

A heartbeat is simply snapping your arms straight forward from the goblet squat position. That cramp between your sternum and belt is called "your abs." I know of no better six-pack exercise, or a better way to teach this feeling of inner pressure.

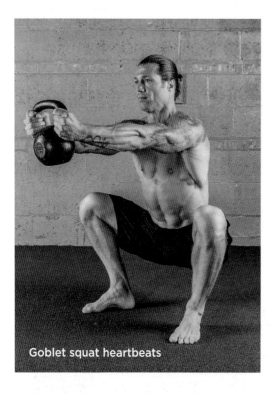

Goblet squat heartbeats

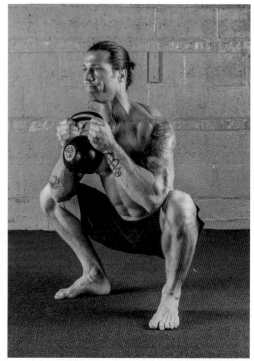

Loaded carries

The loaded carries are basic training for both anaconda strength and arrow training. The suitcase carry—walking with only one side loaded, like carrying a suitcase—is the key to teaching the body to stone up against the forces of a load. Horn walks, walking with the kettlebell held in the goblet squat position, keeps the belly constricted throughout the movement. Heartbeat walks, punching the weight forward while walking, also highlight the body's need to hold and apply pressure.

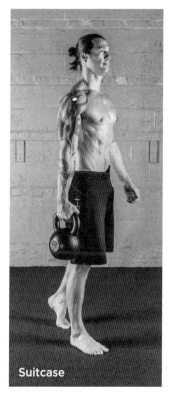
Suitcase

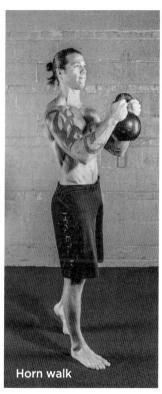
Horn walk

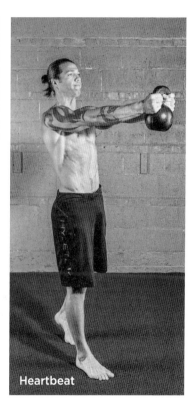
Heartbeat

BODYWEIGHT ROLLING

The get-up (rolling on the ground while loaded) gives us insights into armor building. Of course, any kind of rolling on the ground teaches the athlete how to get back into action ("knocked down six times, get back up seven") and how to toughen up the skin and systems to deal with collisions.

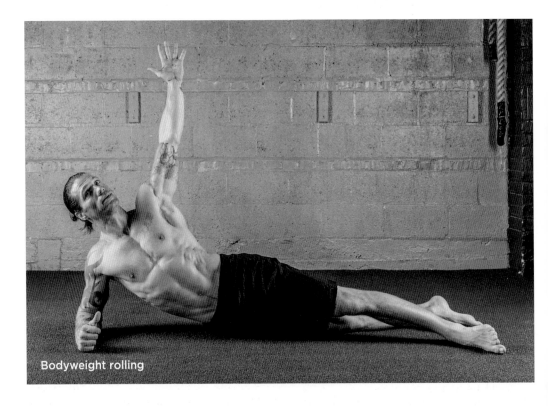
Bodyweight rolling

If you are coaching an athlete or team, match the "stone" training with the needs of the sport. Enough is enough here.

All too often, none is done.

This is Hardstyle: understanding the need for bow, arrow, hammer, and stone. The HKC three provides all of it.

Why the HKC?

Sometimes, when I repeat the same answer to a question more than a few times, I begin to wonder why people even ask me questions.

Exercises for fat loss?
"Sure, swings, goblet squats and get-ups."

Elderly clients?
"Sure, swings, goblet squats and get-ups."

Travel related issues for elite athletes and collision occupations?
"Sure, swings, goblet squats and get-ups."

Most people come to coaches and trainers wanting a magic wand treatment—Harry Potter and the Six Pack Abs—but what they NEED is hip flexor stretching, t-spine mobility, rotary stability and basic movements. They NEED to move, and they NEED to open the hips, spine, and shoulders.

They need the information from the Hardstyle Kettlebell Certification: the swing, goblet squat and get-up.

I have spent my life trying to understand weightlifting. It seems to me that there are three important keys:

- Fundamental Human Movements
- Reps and Sets
- Load

I also think this is the correct order to approach weightlifting. First, we need to establish the correct postures and patterns, then work around a reasonable number of movements in a training session. Finally, we should discuss the load. Sadly, the industry—and I am guilty of this as well—has switched the order and made a 500 pound deadlift the "answer" to improving one's game or cutting some fat.

Also note that I said "training session" as opposed to a workout, because I can work you out:

"Hey, go run to Peru!"
"Hey, go do 50,000 burpees."
"Hey, go swim to Alaska."

But, please don't think those workouts will improve your skill set or your long-term ability to play sports or simply age gracefully.

At the HKC, we learn what I consider to be the key patterns to human movement: the swing, the goblet squat and the get-up. The Hip Displacement Continuum is a term I invented to discuss hip movement. The HDC has two ends: the swing and the goblet squat. The swing demands maximal hip hinge and minimal knee bend while the goblet squat demands maximal hip hinge along with maximal knee bend.

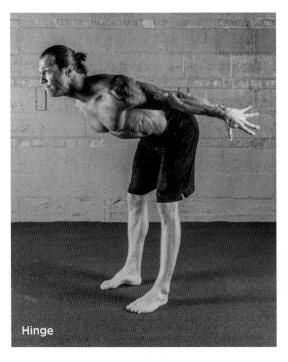

Hinge

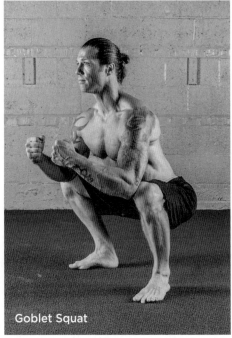

Goblet Squat

The movements are the same but different in their ability to remind the body of the most powerful movements it can perform. The get-up (not the "Turkish sit-up" as I often note) is a one-stop course in the basics of every human movement from rolling and hinging to lunging and locking out.

So, the HKC covers basic human movements in a way that is unlike any other system or school. As I often argue, add the push-up and, honestly, the system might be complete.

Here are the basics of proper training:

1. Training sessions need to be repeatable.
2. Training sessions should put you on the path of progress towards your goals.
3. Training sessions should focus on quality.

What is the key to quality? I have a simple answer for most people: control your repetitions.

In teaching the get-up, or using this wonderful lift as a tool to discover your body, keep the reps "around" ten. Now, you can think about this as a total of ten with five on the right and five on the left, or you can try ten right and ten left. But, please don't make it a war over the numbers. Do the get-ups, feel better and move along.

I have noted that if I do get-ups as part of my warm up along with some get-up drills for "this or that" (the highly technical name we use for correctives), I am sweating and pushing into a "workout" at around ten total reps. Certainly, at times, you can do more.

Week in and week out, think of doing "around" ten reps of the get-up per session.

The goblet squat seems to lock in around 15-25 reps per workout. Later, in the section on programming, I will expand on this insight.

One of the great insights, among many, that I picked up at the RKC is the idea of doing twenty swings with one kettlebell and ten swings with two kettlebells. After doing literally hundreds of swings a day, I noted that my technique held up fine with that ten and twenty range. It is the basic teaching of sports: don't let quantity influence quality. In other words, ten good reps are far better than dozens of crappy reps. If you want more volume, just do more sets.

Of course, there are times when you should do more than twenty reps—there are times when you want to do all kinds of things. Though, most of the time you just need to keep moving ahead. I call these the "Punch the Clock" workouts and I think they are the key to staying in the game.

You may ask if this is enough.

Over time, yes!

It seems that 75-250 swings a day is in the "wheelhouse" for the swing's minimum effective dose. Yes, you can do more, but you want to be able to literally do them day in, day out, year in, and year out.

Finally—and don't take this as a joke—if it is too light, go heavier. And, if you went too heavy, try a lighter kettlebell. Doing a combination of swings and goblet squats with a big kettlebell is a killer workout. But, it is simple to scale a training session up and down by simply changing the kettlebell. Yes, it's that simple. If you look at movement first, then reps, then for whatever reason correct loading seems to make more sense, too.

This is the HKC and I love it. In a one-day course, we learn and do (a lot of "do") the three core movements of the kettlebell world.

THREE MOVEMENTS

The swing, the goblet squat and the get-up are the foundation of the kettlebell world. These three movements alone can challenge strength, power, endurance, mobility and flexibility.

The get-up gets people up and down off the ground and puts great demands on shoulder mobility and stability.

Swings and goblet squats are the two most powerful movements a human can do, and they place a high demand on hip (and leg and back) mobility and stability.

The hips and shoulders are the connecting links between the powerful core and our whippy, fast friends, the arms and the legs. Years ago, at the UCLA RKC Certification, Doctor Mark Cheng explained a key to understanding Chinese Medicine:

The Four Knots

Like a knot on your shoelace, the shoulders and hips have to be both tight and loose. Your shoelace has to be tight enough to keep your shoe on under normal circumstances and loose enough to untie at the end of the day.

The hips and shoulders are the Four Knots. They must be tight enough to stay together under great stress or ballistic forces, yet loose enough to move in a full range of motion.

In addition to tightening and loosening the Four Knots, the Hardstyle Three also provide superior fat loss with the swing, full body tension with the goblet squat, and practically "everything else" with the get-up.

We will discuss the swing and goblet squat first, since these two can be understood similarly, and have some things in common. But in this case, being close—as the old joke goes—only counts with hand grenades.

First, consider the biggest issue with the swing and goblet squat: the Hip Displacement Continuum. The swing is NOT a squat; the squat is NOT a swing. Next, we will introduce the secret of squats and swings, using the glutes (butt) as the key to the movements. After that, we will discuss the practical teaching of both the swing and the squat.

Let's clear up some confusion first.

The Hip Displacement Continuum

Breon Hole was struggling with her kettlebell swing. Josh Vert asked me to help, as Breon's lower back would scream after a few repetitions of the swing. Within two reps, I stopped her.

It's funny because years ago, a young man told me that squats hurt his knees. I asked him to demonstrate his squat. He did, and I said, "Squats don't hurt your knees; whatever you were doing there hurts your knees."

I told Breon, "Swings don't hurt your back; whatever the hell you are doing hurts your back."

Ah, Great coaching again! I knew something was wrong and stated the obvious. Breon then asked the million-dollar question, "Well, then, what am I doing wrong?"

Thank you, Breon. You see, I could SEE the problem, but I had no ability to fix it. Oh, I knew drills and we could have pushed, pulled and prodded her to a better movement, but I knew that I didn't know what to do.

I knew that Breon was swinging incorrectly. But, I didn't know much else. Usually, we would wave our hands around, do some drills, and then through sheer luck, fix her swing. But, I knew we would still be missing something.

She was bending her knees too much which let the kettlebell go too low. This tossed all the forces onto her lower back. What she was doing is sometimes called the "squatting swing."

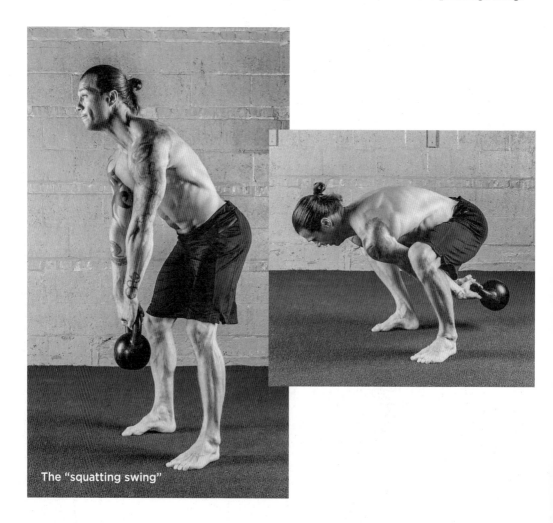

The "squatting swing"

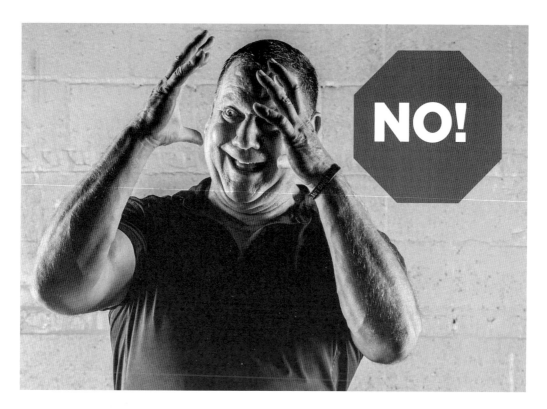

When I first said "squatting swing" out loud, my little world of lifting came into absolute focus.

The swing is not a squat.   **The squat is not a swing.**

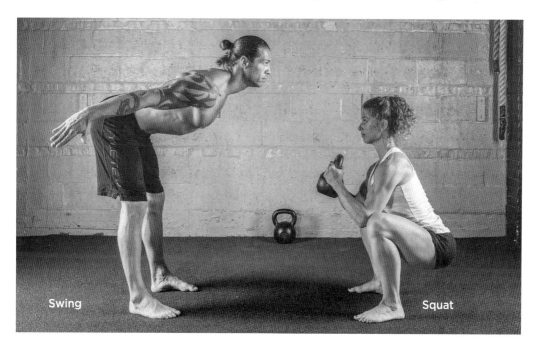

It is the greatest insight of my teaching career. We went to a white board and began talking about this notion. It soon became known as the Hip Displacement Continuum. This is the original picture and the notes are from an email I sent Mark Twight (founder of Gym Jones and the legendary trainer of the movie *300*):

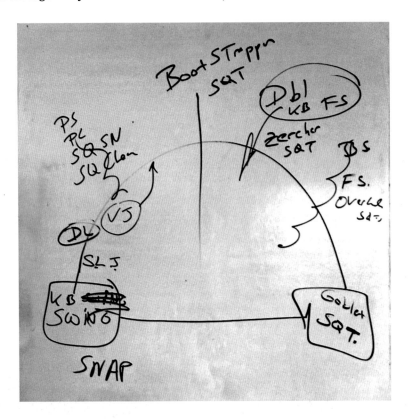

Breon and Josh Vert asked a good question.

Breon was taught to do swings from a "deep squat" and that "you are cheating if you don't deep squat". Well, no...

Put this on a "rainbow" curve or continuum.

On the far left:
- Vertical Jump
- Standing Long Jump
- Swings (all variations)
- Romanian Deadlifts
- Tackling in football would also go here

In the middle:
- Bootstrapper Squat

In a narrow beam:
- Snatches
- Cleans
- Deadlifts
- Back Squats
- Front Squats
- Overhead Squats

On the far right:
- Goblet Squats

The most powerful movements the human body can achieve are from the swing position or, as it has been called more recently, the hinge movement. If you are walking and a rattlesnake crosses your path, your "leap" away will be more on the left side of the continuum. If you wish to kiss the rattler first, then that movement would be a squat.

You decide: leap away from the rattler or kiss the rattler?

Bad jumpers start with a lot of knee bend and diminish the pop of the hinging hips. Bad squatters bend their knees a lot and ignore the hip movement. The continuum clarified this thinking for me. Forever. It was one of the few times that some mental effort actually improved physical performance.

As a test, we tried a series of standing long jump tests. First, we encouraged the athlete to use a lot of knee bend and told them to "really use your legs" then tested three jumps. Next, we asked for nearly no knee bend, but a snappy hip movement. Most athletes came within three inches of their best jump with this style, and many athletes actually did better. Finally, we allowed some additional knee bend, but emphasized the explosive hip, for the athlete's last few attempts. It was more common than not for them to reach personal records during this final test.

"Hinge" movements, like the swing have a deep hip movement and minimal knee bend. Squat movements have deep movements in both the hips and the knees.

So, memorize this:

- **Hinge (swings, jumps):** deep hip movement, minimal knee movement.
- **Squats:** deep hip movement, deep knee movement.

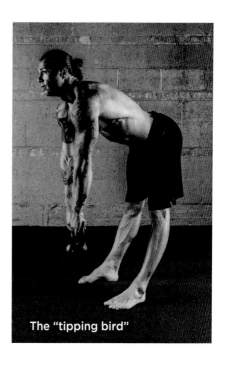

The "tipping bird"

In hinge/swing movements, you might note that the knee bends more and more, but there is always some bend. There always needs to be a slight bend in the knees during any movement. A stiff-legged swing is known as "The Tipping Bird," like those old bar standards where the plastic bird swings back and forth into a drink. One of the great errors of beginning squatters is to lock out the knees at the start or top of the movement. No need to jack up your knees for life, my friend, keep a slight bend in the knees.

It is interesting to think about the popularity of leg extension and leg curl machines in the Seventies and Eighties. These movements have deep knee bends, but technically no hip involvement. Some research has indicated that these movements are terrible for the knees. Mother Nature seems to know best when it comes to training.

When someone complains that swings hurt their back, it is often because they have turned the movement into a "squatting swing". Always keep the kettlebell above the knees, "attack the zipper," hinge the hips, make the hips fold—or use whatever clue that will help you. When someone complains that squats hurt their knees, take a moment to check their hips.

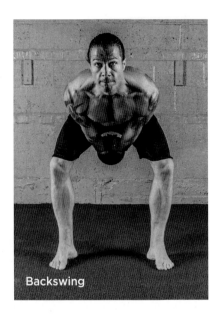
Backswing

GLUTEAL AMNESIA

I often joke to my audience and say, "You are sitting on a goldmine." The glutes might be the most important muscles in the body, but until recently, many have ignored this muscle family. The glutes are the foundation of power and the fountain of youth. Healthy glutes show the world you are young, vibrant and virile.

This isn't hyperbole: there is a wonderful scene in *Sex and the City* where a very wealthy man—with a lot of Viagra—loses the girl because of his saggy bottom. Droopy butt cheeks seem to denote weakness, illness and injury. The inability to tightly flex the glutes has become so common that Stu McGill, the noted Canadian back specialist, has come up with a great term for this condition: gluteal amnesia.

The inability to hold one's belt line at a position parallel to the floor is the first sign of gluteal amnesia. I first heard about this concept decades ago in the work of Laurence Morehouse and Leonard Gross. In their books, especially *Total Fitness* and *Maximum Performance*, there is a small point made about how effortlessly one woman glides across the campus. Her belt line is parallel to the ground as she moves. The authors compare this to how most people allow their belt lines to angle downward. The cure for this is to squeeze the butt cheeks.

Stand and try to give yourself a flat belt line: Squeeze your cheeks hard together. If you find that the front of your hips begins to complain about a stretch, you might have gluteal amnesia. If you can't figure out how to squeeze your cheeks, you might have a nice case of gluteal amnesia.

Imagine that the pelvis is a bowl with water in it—and you want to keep the bowl from dripping or pouring water out. Most Americans are pouring water out of the front. If you think of the rib cage as a box, you want to keep the "box on the bowl." If the bowl is calm and quiet, the box can happily sit on it for generations.

If you tilt the bowl forward, something in the body will have to work overtime and this often leads to back issues, tight hip flexors and the dreaded belly pooch.

At the top of a swing and the top of a goblet squat, your belt should be parallel with the floor. And, yes, coaching can be that simple.

In total honesty, I have been there. Years ago, my necrotic left hip was slowly destroying my ability to walk, train and live. Weeks before my total hip replacement surgery, I noticed an odd thing, I couldn't squeeze my left butt cheek. I couldn't "find it."

Mike Warren Brown, the Director of Programming at my gym, spends most of his time working with elderly clients. Training older clients is a window into the entire population: some of us are aging well and some of us are not. Mike has a simple drill to "find" the glutes.

Lay on the floor. (For some elderly clients, just getting to the floor will highlight their issues with age and disuse.) Slip your hands under your butt cheeks (cue the usual joke, "I said YOUR butt cheeks") and consciously squeeze the left and right glutes into your hands.

This might seem like an exercise for just geriatric patients. But, here's the thing—if you CRAMP a hamstring during a hip thrust or any other member of the glute training exercise family, then well, to channel Jeff Foxworthy, "You might just have glute amnesia."

> ## PAY ATTENTION
> If you do lots of swings and serious glute work, I WANT your hamstrings to be sore the next day or so. As I often tell people, "If your lower back hurts after swings, you are not listening and you are doing them wrong. If your hamstrings hurt, I'm a great coach."

We are not talking about a hamstring feeling sore a day or two from now, we are looking at hamstrings cramping while doing the glute movement. The "cure" is often Mike's "Butt Awareness Drill" (BAD...copyright pending). Lay on the ground, cup your butt cheeks and practice controlling the squeeze.

Back in the 1980s, we did pelvic tilts at the Olympic Training Center and I thought they looked stupid. As so often happens, I walked away from one of the best exercises ever invented for teaching people to use their glutes and for overall athletic improvement. Today, we refer to pelvic tilts as hip thrusts and we can all thank Bret Contreras for making them part of the general training discussion.

I teach these with the thumbs driving into the ground, as pictured. It is like the top of the swing, but on the ground. The reason I teach hip thrusts with the hands like this is to keep people from doing more work with their shoulders rounded forward in the "staring at the computer screen" position. I want their shoulders back and packed and this little tweak helps a lot.

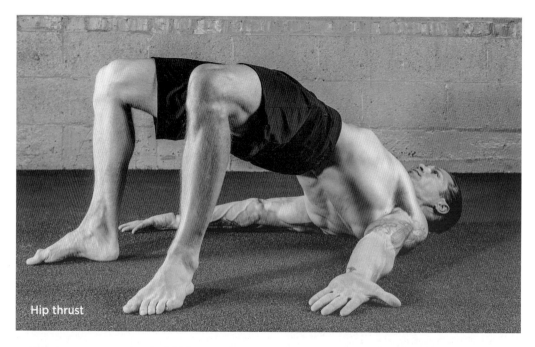

Hip thrust

Hip thrusts are great held like planks, or you can choose to do them for reps. For the record, if someone wants a video of what a hip thrust plank (or gluteal bridge, or supine bridge) looks like, simply look at the picture above and imagine the athlete not moving for thirty seconds or so. (Attempt at humor: I was once asked for a video of an isometric move pictured on an article. I'm still not sure what the person wanted, because a video without movement and a picture are pretty much the same thing.)

The hip thrust can be done with bodyweight, bands, or with loads like kettlebells or barbells. The hip thrust is the start of the famous "Buns and Guns" workout we have at our gym.

QUICK POINT

Like most strength coaches, I have rarely worried about programming arm work or bench presses for my male athletes or abdominal work for my female athletes as they tend to happily do this on their own time. But, since the buns part of this workout is so intense, we add biceps and triceps work at the end as a bit of dessert. And, it works. Yummy.

Our gym's basic "Buns" workout:

- Hip thrusts up to 25 reps (We used much higher reps, but 20-25 work the "best")
- Squat variation for 10 reps
- Swing variation (heavy) for 15 reps
- Mini-band walks with the bands around the socks for as far as possible in each direction

Mike Warren Brown added a key point to every focused glute workout: hip flexor stretches. Hip flexor stretches should be done during the rest periods, and most people will know a few variations of this movement.

His argument, and Vlad Janda would agree, is that the hip flexors are pulling the pelvic bowl forward as we get more and more turned into a comma shape from constantly sitting. Since the glute work is actively prying the hip flexors, let's give the flexors a chance to really unlock during the stretching periods.

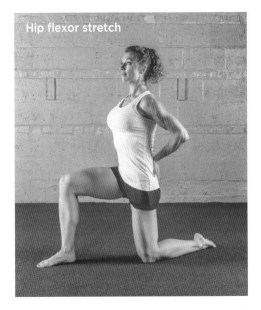

Hip flexor stretch

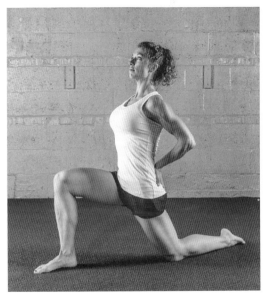

After the buns workout and hip flexor stretches, it's not unusual for people to say something like, "My back feels so much better." Getting the box on the bowl releases the stresses on the back.

During the mini-band walks, keep side-stepping and reaching as far as you can with the lead foot. It also helps to step "heel first" as you push sideways. The lead heel leads the whole body. There is a delicious cramping feeling in the outer, upper glutes indicating that you are indeed working the right area.

Once again:
- Hip Thrust
- Squat
- Swing
- Mini-Band Walk (if applicable)
- RKC Hip Flexor Stretch

The devil is in the details, but goblet squats make an easier workout than double kettlebell front squats. I find that the squat tends to cascade pain and anguish into the other moves. Using the thighs to push the tired glutes along is certainly nothing new, but this workout seems to be a "one stop shop" to fix the glutes and gluteal amnesia.

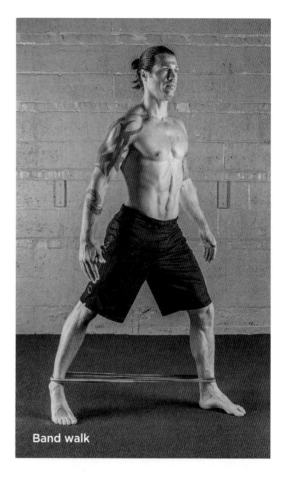
Band walk

It is possible to do the workout for up to four rounds, but generally most people find that two rounds are repeatable and doable week in and week out. This workout can be done twice a week as part of a general training program. Oddly, it doesn't take very much time. Strive to move from exercise to exercise as quickly as you can.

For a pure kettlebell glute challenge, we can fall back on this classic:

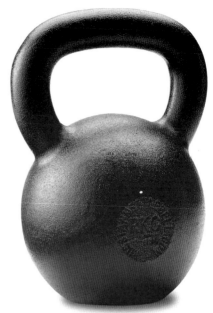

10 Swings / 10 Goblet Squats
9 Swings / 9 Goblet Squats
8 Swings / 8 Goblet Squats
7 Swings / 7 Goblet Squats
6 Swings / 6 Goblet Squats
5 Swings / 5 Goblet Squats
4 Swings / 4 Goblet Squats
3 Swings / 3 Goblet Squats
2 Swings / 2 Goblet Squats
1 Swing / 1 Goblet Squat

That's 55 reps of each movement. Ideally, one does not put the kettlebell down and finishes each and every rep with cramped glutes at the top positions.

I'm a strength coach, so my approach to gluteal amnesia is lifting and stretching. My answer to a lot of things is lifting and stretching. Some people and some clients may have issues that need surgical intervention or specific therapies. But, for most people, focusing on training the glutes hard will be the single best thing they can do for all conditions and qualities, including elite performance.

Finally, because I KNOW someone will ask, the "Guns" part of the "Buns and Guns" program is two to four supersets of curls and triceps work to build my "Arm-acondas", pythons, or guns.

FOUR SQUARE:
THE NON-BALLISTIC HINGES

I teach the pelvic tilt (hip thrust) to death. I teach a variety of corrections and correctives in teaching the hinge to people who have lost their hinge. Suddenly, the phrase "unhinged" has a whole new meaning.

But, there comes a time when we need to get the trainee on their feet and hinging with load.

Let me give you a warning: never add speed to poor movement. Don't go fast through dysfunction.

I make a joke when I explain this, and it is a joke. I hope you understand I am using hyperbole to make a point:

"When I drink really heavily, I like to drive as fast as I can so I can get home quicker and not be a menace on the road."

Nearly everyone sees the idiocy behind this statement—nearly. In the world of teaching the swing, if we have poor movement, twisting or buckling versus hinging, adding speed will probably take a few pieces of bone, cartilage and ligament with it.

Sadly, we see this all the time. It is much better to progress slowly with load. In this case, "slowly" means having the patience to take weeks and months to learn the swing before increasing the speed of movement in training.

I use four different load positions to teach the hinge. Each has pros and cons—some people love one and hate the other. In my experience, having all four tools is better than settling on one. A full coaching toolbox filled with a variety of answers is often better than praying for the "one size fits all" extreme.

KETTLEBELL DEADLIFT FROM A BOX

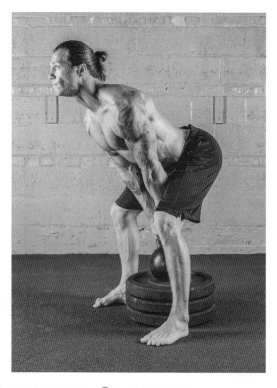

For most people, doing a kettlebell deadlift from the floor quickly turns into something more like a sumo squat or plié from ballet. Instead, we want to stretch the hamstrings and make the person "hinge." For most people, raising the kettlebell up by placing it on a box, bench or plate will position the kettlebell so that the body hinges in and out as the kettlebell raises up and down.

I err on the side of "too high" in the beginning. Just reaching back between the thighs and gripping the kettlebell can be a great teaching moment for many clients.

Waiter Bow

This time, grip the kettlebell by the horns and place the handle on the back of the neck. This starting position should look like the beginning of a kettlebell French press. Now, push the butt back with the knees slightly bent, and "bow" forward under control. Focus on how the hamstrings are stretching and loading. When you can't go BACK any more, snap up into a vertical plank.

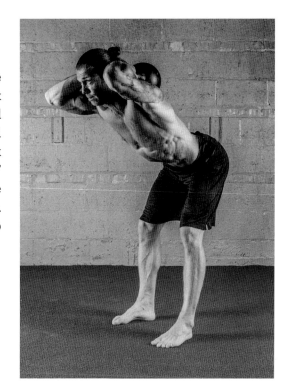

The RDL Hinge

I met Nico Vlad, the inventor of the Romanian deadlift, and I watched him do them. Those who argue that he didn't might not have been there that day. I always listen to Olympic gold medalists when it comes to training. The RDL hinge is simple. Hold the kettlebell by the handle BEHIND the back. Push your butt straight back into the kettlebell until you feel the hamstrings stretch. Continue to push this stretch until you can't! Fold over or bend the knees more, then snap up into a vertical plank using the hamstrings like the bowstring of a bow and arrow.

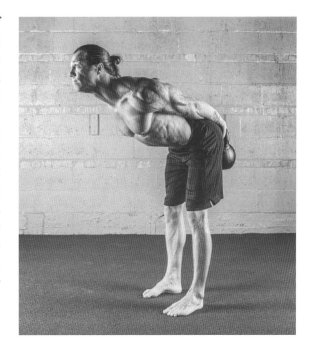

THE BULGARIAN GOAT BAG SWING

I came up with this drill while working with Josh Vert. We were trying to make the swing easier and easier to learn. The name was our way of having fun while trying to poke at some people who take all of this a bit too seriously.

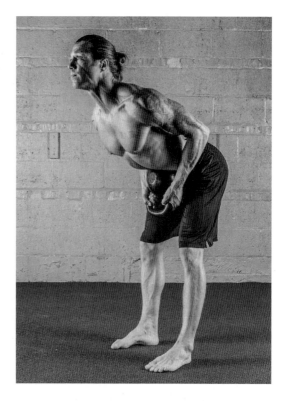

The Bulgarian goat bag swing is simple. Hold the kettlebell by the horns in a curl grip and put the base of the kettlebell on your ab wall (below the sternum and xiphoid process). One key to a perfect swing is finishing with the abs tight, so having a piece of iron on top of them naturally tightens everything up! Push the hips back, stretch the hammies, then snap back up to the vertical plank.

THE ORIGINAL BUTT BLASTER 5000

10 Bulgarian Goat Bag Swings / 10 Goblet Squats
9 Bulgarian Goat Bag Swings / 9 Goblet Squats
8 Bulgarian Goat Bag Swings / 8 Goblet Squats
7 Bulgarian Goat Bag Swings / 7 Goblet Squats
6 Bulgarian Goat Bag Swings / 6 Goblet Squats
5 Bulgarian Goat Bag Swings / 5 Goblet Squats
4 Bulgarian Goat Bag Swings / 4 Goblet Squats
3 Bulgarian Goat Bag Swings / 3 Goblet Squats
2 Bulgarian Goat Bag Swings / 2 Goblet Squats
1 Bulgarian Goat Bag Swing / 1 Goblet Squat

This remains one of the best teaching workouts for discerning the Hip Displacement Continuum, and for discovering the glutes.

SWINGS

Just as I began my first workouts in 1965, an interesting exercise was slowly slipping away from the gyms, weight rooms and spas of the world: the swing. As the era of Universal and Nautilus machines pushed kettlebells, fixed barbells and gymnastics equipment from the floor, one of the best overall "fat burning athlete builders" also disappeared. Many European and Australian coaches continued using swings in their training programs, but basically the movement went the way of Nehru Jackets (this is the 1960s) in the United States.

Then something amazing happened. Pavel Tsatsouline and John Du Cane brought kettlebells and kettlebell training back in the early 2000s. If you have seen a kettlebell, you have them to thank for it. If you know someone certified to teach kettlebells, they owe those two a letter of thanks. The swing is so popular now that monthly 10,000 swing challenges appear on social media as often as memes with sarcastic Willy Wonka.

Sadly, swings are very easy to do incorrectly. Let's go through a short list here to make your swing better and help you not look like an idiot...or worse.

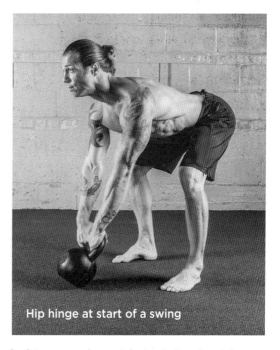

Hip hinge at start of a swing

1. The swing is a hip hinge snapping into a plank. Nearly every problem comes from missing this point. When you hinge, your hips bend maximally, but your knees only bend minimally. In other words, don't squat your swing! (The squat is both hips and knees bending maximally).

2. After a swing workout, you should feel sore in your hamstrings, although I will allow that your butt may be sore, too. If you feel it in your lower back, you are doing it wrong! Wrong. Generally, people who swing into a sore back are not hinging. The weight should be aimed at your zipper and you should wisely let it miss. In the hinge, reach straight back deeply with your arms like you are deep snapping to a punter.

3. The top of a swing brings you to a vertical plank. Your shoulders should be packed down (no shrugging at all), your butt cheeks and quads should be squeezing, your lats should be tight and your feet should be pushing straight down. The kettlebell doesn't have to come very high (it is okay to "float" a bit). When swinging with a heavy kettlebell, it might not get up to your belt height. The crown of your head should stretch straight up to its zenith and you should look like you are planking on the ground (except that you are standing).

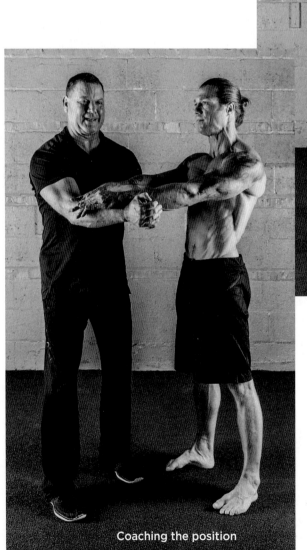

Top of swing

Coaching the position

4. Don't TRY to be stupid with swings. Keep your eyes locked in one place. I recommend "eyes on horizon" or find a spot on the wall that would basically be the same height and keep looking at it throughout the move. NEVER look down or, worse, back—even if the person telling you to do this compromising position is extremely famous.

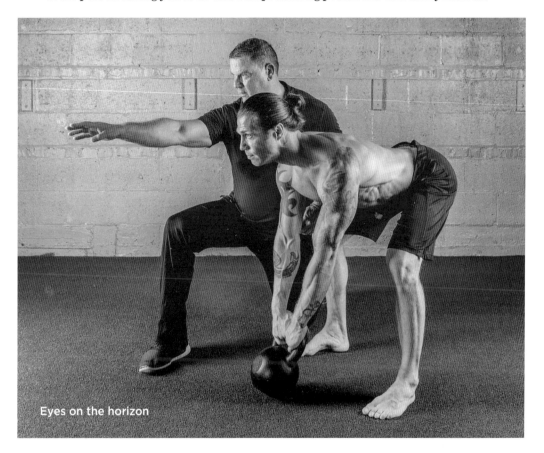

Eyes on the horizon

5. The swing is all about generating a lot of power in each stroke. So, hinge and explode (like a tackle in football), snap into the plank and then throw the kettlebell back at your zipper. The swing is different from its cousin the snatch in one simple way—when doing the kettlebell snatch you are thinking of throwing the kettlebell upwards, like the Highland Games Weight Over Bar event. In the swing, it helps to think about throwing the kettlebell forward (think it, don't do it). Occasionally, I have actually had people throw the kettlebell when learning swings just so they get the sense of this violent move.

6. For most of us, the two-handed swing is going to be enough. Moving to one hand swings has a great value for grip strength and cardiovascular work, but all too often, people twist and sway with this one-handed movement. Yes, I would love for you to do it correctly, but if you can't get competent coaching, stick with the two-hand swing.

7. Swings work very well with a variety of repetition schemes. Although we start each workout with five sets of fifteen swings (followed by goblet squats, marching in place, then a flexibility move), we rarely do the same rep scheme back to back. The following are two variations that work well and have been well tested by my group and myself with 40,000 swings (four runs through the 10,000-swing challenge).

Variation One:
10 Swings
15 Swings
25 Swings
50 Swings

The fifty reps are tough, but the nice thing about this variation is that when you've completed it, you have just done one hundred swings. Do this variation five times and well, you can do the math. Once again, the fifty reps are tough.

Variation Two:
15 Swings
35 Swings

We moved to this variation after realizing that fifty swings five times a day, five days a week for four weeks was really hard. So, this little compromise gives us an easier set followed by a harder set. It's fifty quick reps and we like to mix in strength and flexibility movements between each round.

You can certainly do any combination, but we tested many variations and these two worked best.

"Most of the time," is a dangerous phrase. I would suggest keeping your swing reps in the range of either ten or fifteen per set. Then stick to this number as much as you can to minimize confusion.

8. Do NOT practice the style of swings where the arms go above the head. Just snap the kettlebell forward and somewhere between belt height and shoulder height (as long as the crown of the head is driving to its zenith), then actively toss the kettlebell back to the zipper. "Zipper to zenith" might be a coaching cue to consider.

9. Pick up the kettlebell "like a professional" and finish the set in the same way. Every set, I spend time getting my feet positioned and firm, then I hinge back, tighten the lats, and finally find my focus point on the horizon. After finishing a set, put the kettlebell down while maintaining your back position and strive for a quiet landing on the ground. I like no sound at all, actually.

10. Finally, I use the swing in warm ups, athletic prep, and general training for all populations. If you want to do them correctly, hire an HKC or RKC certified kettlebell instructor. There are plenty of regressions and corrections that can be added to your program to clean up your movement, but no article or video is as good as hands-on coaching. Obviously, I believe that for all training ideas, too. When I first learned the swing, I hired someone to walk me through the basics and it was worth every dime.

Hopefully, the swing is here to stay. It remains dear to all of us who want a simple, effective training tool that addresses so many issues. Swing away.

THE GOBLET SQUAT

The greatest impact I've had on strength and conditioning starts with a story. Years ago, when faced with 400 athletes who couldn't squat correctly, I attempted to teach the squat, move after move, lift after lift.

I failed each and every time.

I saw glimmers of hope when teaching one kid the Zercher squat (weight held in the crooks of the elbows…enjoy). A few athletes picked up the pattern when we lifted kettlebells off the ground by the ball, a move we called "potato sack squats" since it looks like we're picking a sack of potatoes up from the ground. But nothing was working.

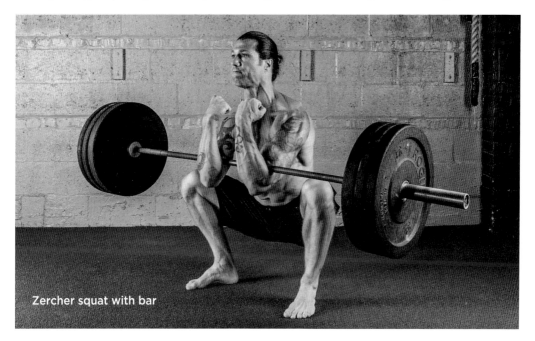
Zercher squat with bar

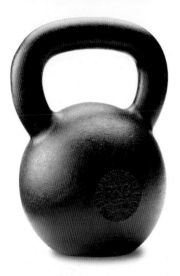

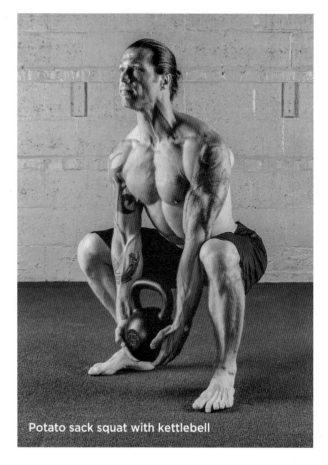

Potato sack squat with kettlebell

Somewhere between a Zercher and a potato sack squat was the answer.

It came to me when I was resting between swings and holding the weight in front of me like I was holding the Holy Grail. I squatted down from there, pushed my knees out with my elbows and... behold, the goblet squat!

Yes, the squat is that easy. It's a basic human movement and you just have to be reminded how to do it.

Squats can do more for total muscle mass and overall body strength than probably all the other lifts combined. Likewise, doing squats incorrectly can do more damage than probably all the other moves, too.

Let's start simple. Find a place where no one is watching and squat down. At the bottom of the squat, the deepest you can go, push your knees out with your elbows. Relax...and go a bit deeper. Your feet should be flat on the floor. For the bulk of the population, this small movement—driving your knees out with your elbows—will simplify squatting forever.

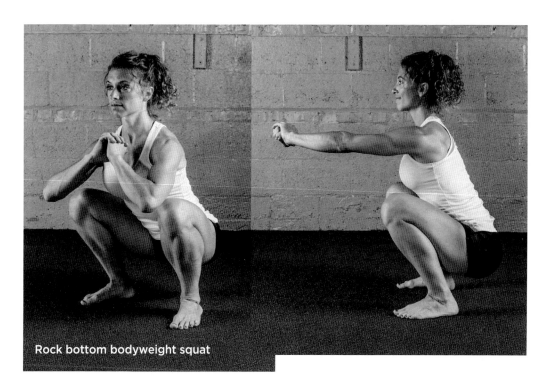
Rock bottom bodyweight squat

Next, try this little drill. Stand arms-length away from a door knob. Grab the door knob with both hands and get your chest up. Up? Imagine being on a California beach when a swimsuit model walks by. When I have an athlete do this, he will immediately puff up his chest, which tightens the lower back and locks the whole upper body. The lats naturally spread a bit and the shoulders come back a little, too.

Now, lower yourself down.

What people discover at this instant is a basic physiological fact. The legs are not stuck like stilts under the torso. Rather, the torso is slung between the legs. As you go down, leaning back with straight arms, you'll discover one of the true keys of lifting: You squat between your legs.

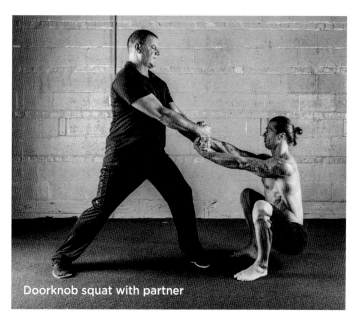
Doorknob squat with partner

THE HARDSTYLE KETTLEBELL CHALLENGE

You do not fold and unfold like an accordion—you sink between your legs.

Don't just sit and read this. Do it!

Now you're ready to learn the single best lifting movement of all time—the goblet squat. Grab a kettlebell by the horns (like you're holding a goblet) and hold it against your chest.

You see—goblet squats.

With the weight cradled against your chest, squat down with the goal of sliding your elbows past the insides of your knees. Your elbows are pointed down, and it's okay to have them push against your knees—pushing your knees out as you descend.

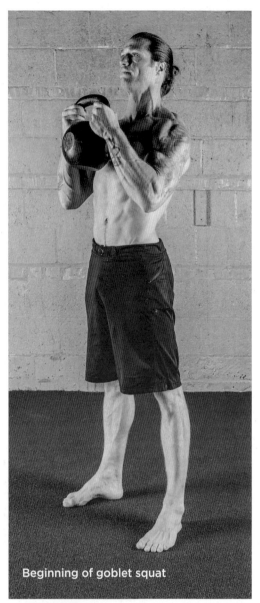

Beginning of goblet squat

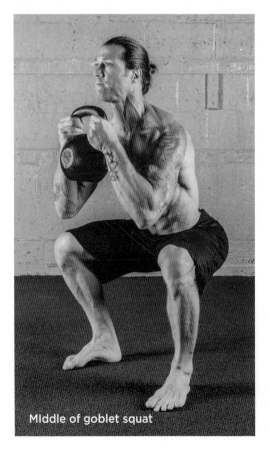

Middle of goblet squat

This is the big-money key to learning movements in the gym—let the body teach the body what to do. Listen to this: Try to stay out of it! Thinking through a movement often leads to problems; let the elbows glide down by touching the inner knees and good things will happen.

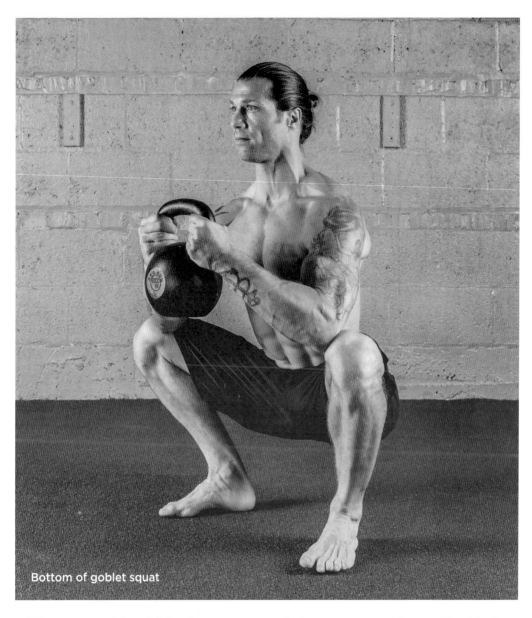

Bottom of goblet squat

The more an athlete thinks, the more we can find ways to screw things up. Don't believe me? Join a basketball team and get into a crucial situation. Shoot a one-and-one with three seconds to go, down by two points, and get back to me later if you decided thinking was a good idea.

I'm not sure I should tell you this, but here it is: I think goblet squats are all the squatting most people need. Seriously, once you grab a kettlebell over one hundred pounds and do a few sets of ten goblet squats, you might wonder how the toilet got so low the next morning.

As a simple guide for foot placement, do three consecutive vertical jumps, then look down. This is roughly where to place your feet every time you squat. You know that the toes should be out a little, and most people look down and see their toes are magically out. You don't want to go completely east and west here, but you do want some toe turn out.

There is an important coaching point to note: the goblet squat and all the drills I've described teach patterning. Unless you have the pattern, you shouldn't move into heavier work. Until a person can prove they have the stability, flexibility and, most importantly, the patterning of the goblet squat, don't worry excessively about load...or even trying other squatting movements.

The more I work, however, the more I am convinced that the goblet squat is all most of us will ever need.

The Get-Up
Looking Back on Rolling Around

As the 1960s were coming to a close, my family—like many working families—was struggling with the pressures of Vietnam Vets in our house, social strife and the looming fear of a Nuclear War. Not every minute of my youth was a Norman Rockwell painting and just mentioning Rockwell might have just aged me a bit.

At the same time, I was beginning to realize that I wanted to be an athlete. My family, of course, was extremely athletic. But, I wanted to do something no one in my family did—I wanted to play football. I wandered over to the Orange Library and found a book on football. It was Eliot Asinof's *Seven Days to Sunday* and I read about a linebacker named Kenny Avery.

As a small segue, I also spotted *The Sword in the Stone* by T. H. White on the "recommended" shelf. It's funny to think that 45 years later these two books still impact my thinking and life choices. The title of my best seller, *Never Let Go*, comes from White's book. I checked out both books then went home and read them cover to cover. And then, I read them again.

Avery threw the discus, so I threw the discus. Avery lifted weights and did gymnastics. I knew a little about weights, but I saw the gap in my knowledge. So, I went back to the library and picked up Myles Callum's book, *Body-Building and Self-Defense*. I followed Callum's advice religiously. I learned the lifts, the falls, the tumbles and the basics of self-defense.

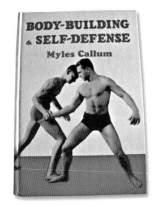

Not long ago, Callum's book was sitting on the shelf in my gym and Brian Deede, former Ball State linebacker and all around good guy, picked it up. Like most people, he snickered at the guys training in just gym shorts and asked me if the book had value today. We flipped through it again and decided that if you cut and pasted the words, updated the pictures with guys with tats and board shorts and called it "Strength Training for MMA", we would have a best seller.

The book came out in 1962 and is still pretty good. Much of the advice stands the test of time. "If you don't want to get hurt, learn to fall." Callum's advice on dealing with a robber with a gun is still pretty good: it is better to lose 100% of your money than take that one percent chance of losing your life.

In 1997, Ken Shamrock came out with *Inside the Lion's Den*. Based on training in the early years of submission fighting, this book deals more with fighting inside the "safe" confines of the fighting cage. In real life fighting, there are no tap outs or referees.

Callum and Shamrock share many of the same core concepts. Callum reflects the total body movements of the 1960s with squats on the toes, Jefferson lifts, and side bends. Shamrock thins the barbell work to simply the bench press, squats, clean and jerks, and curls. But, he also demands high volume of bodyweight squats, tumbling work (both include cartwheels) and something he calls "scrambling," which includes a variety of ground-based exercises and various movement games.

In the 35 years since the publication of these books, we have regressed in the field of fitness, conditioning, and strength work. The influence of the machines, from the Universal Gyms, Nautilus, and all of the knock-offs, had people starting to think in body parts. Then, with the rise of bodybuilding (especially after Arnold's *The Education of a Bodybuilder*) the pump, the blitz and the pythons overtook traditional training.

So, today we now have coaches who specialize in corrective work to undo the problems of their training programs. That was a mean statement, but understand my point—if you are spending more time with foam rolling, rehab, hot tub, massage and other modalities than you are in training, something is very wrong.

Let's just take foam rolling. I often wish someone would just take it away, but I understand why we're doing it. But, an alternative to foam rolling is.... rolling! Shoulder rolls on a wrestling mat not only prep us for life's slips and falls, but has the added benefit of rubbing fascia with a lot of load. Cartwheels are part of my loaded carry family. A cartwheel is literally a moving plank and a great way to check in on your body connections.

The get-up can be a boon for helping people remember how to get up and down from the floor. Pat Flynn regards the get-up as a loaded carry and I think he gets it right. The get-up is a loaded carry with the extra benefit of teaching you to reorient yourself with the floor.

Get-ups combined with Shamrock's "scrambles" would be a fun and enlightening workout for anyone. The scrambles are children's games like leap frog and jumping over sticks. While these are rarely seen in most gyms, they're a lot of fun to do and to coach.

Let me add just one extra thing: Phil Maffetone remarked that 28,000 Americans in my age range die from falls and fall related injuries every year. God forbid you bring peanut butter to a school, but NOTHING serious is being done about fall prevention.

Let me make a small point: recently, the BBC had a show about risks. Eating bacon every day for breakfast might affect your chances of survival the next ten years. How much? The show noted that daily bacon consumption will move you from five in a thousand chance of death to SIX in one thousand.

What's the most dangerous thing you do each day? It might be taking a shower. Day in and day out, my life teeters on entering and exiting my shower. It's the riskiest thing I do as I don't commute to work.

The years of fall training in Judo probably lower my risks. I know how to fall and break a fall. Do your parents know how to fall and recover? Do you?

As nice as it is to have six pack abs, it is also nice to be alive at your grandkid's wedding. So, barf less at your next workout and practice falling. And—like me—be aware of stepping in and out of the shower.

When the running and jogging craze emerged in the late 1960s and 1970s, Ken Cooper reinvented the term "aerobics." Along with all the junk mileage came injuries. The answer was stretching. Static stretching, dynamic stretching, dynamic mobility, and PNF were all touted as the answers to various shin, knee, foot, and hip injuries. Barefoot running has been called the answer lately, too. But there used to be a better approach: stretching in conjunction with proper training.

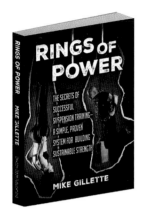

Both Callum and Shamrock discuss flexibility and mobility, but in the classic sense that they are synergistic with the rest of training. Some movements like goblet squats, swings, and windmills simply stretch you out. They are my "go to" movements for blending strength with mobility. You can easily argue for many more. Many movements in the bodyweight world demand flexibility and I have noticed great changes since following the simple advice in the book *Rings of Power*.

Being flexible is important, but being flexible and strong is more important.

For aerobic work or "cardio" (and lo, how I loathe those terms), doing garbage mileage on the track, treadmill, rowing machine and the bicycle certainly have great value... they prepare you for garbage mileage. Shamrock demands 500 bodyweight squats BEFORE he allows you condition with him! Training to fight is not the same as spinning your wheels... literally.

Much can be learned from self-defense and the fighting arts. You don't need to get into the Octagon to learn these lessons. You can get some benefits just by adding get-ups, goblet squats, swings and windmills to your training. You can follow Callum and Shamrock's advice to pare things down and keep things simple.

Fifty plus years from now, you will be more right than wrong.

The Basics of Ground Work

One of the best pieces of equipment you own is literally at your feet. Few seem to use it anymore, but for safety, cardiovascular conditioning and sports improvement, I can't think of a better tool to use.

It is the "ground."

Only rarely do you see people training on the floor anymore. Sure, you might see crunches or foam rolling, but most trainees seem to have some aversion to groundwork. As Maffetone taught us, 28,000 Americans die each year from fall and fall related injuries. I believe that some level of break fall training should be taught in youth as well as a full complement of tumbling. Mastering what to do after you slip is better learned early than too late.

Oddly, the greatest boon from groundwork seems to be getting the heart to start pounding. Adding something as simple as a set of bird dogs to any standard upper body movement will raise the heart rate. I often combine push-ups with squats or swings for this very reason. Yes, swings raise the pulse, but popping up and down from the floor makes it jump even higher.

Moreover, collision sports often come down to this: get knocked down twice, get up three times. In football, the game is often decided after the contact. We now keep stats on "yards after contact." If a defender pops up off the ground and gets back into the play, it will be very hard to make those Xs and Os work on the chalkboard.

GET BACK UPS

I have a little tool to warm up my people and practice groundwork—I call it a "GetBackUp". It's easy to add into any program.

***There's an important key to using this drill: do not over-coach it.
In fact, intentionally under-coach the whole movement.***

Announce the position on the ground (on the front, on the right side, on the left side, push-up position plank, or on the back). Wait for the client, or clients, to get in position. When they have all stopped moving, say, "Get back up." When everyone is standing still, move to the next position.

Series One *(The hands are free)*

- Down on your front (or on your belly)
- Get back up
- Down on your right side
- Get back up
- Down on your left side
- Get back up
- Push-up position plank
- Get back up
- Down on your back
- Get back up

Series Two *(The right hand is stuck to the right knee—tell them a puppy dies if their hands come loose from their knees.)*

- Down on your front (or on your belly)
- Get back up
- Down on your right side
- Get back up
- Down on your left side
- Get back up
- Push-up position plank
- Get back up
- Down on your back
- Get back up

Series Three *(The left hand is stuck to the left knee)*

- Down on your front (or on your belly)
- Get back up
- Down on your right side
- Get back up
- Down on your left side
- Get back up
- Push-up position plank
- Get back up
- Down on your back
- Get back up

Series Four *(The right hand is stuck to the left knee)*

- Down on your front (or on your belly)
- Get back up
- Down on your right side
- Get back up
- Down on your left side
- Get back up
- Push-up position plank
- Get back up
- Down on your back
- Get back up

Series Five *(The left hand is stuck to the right knee)*

- Down on your front (or on your belly)
- Get back up
- Down on your right side
- Get back up
- Down on your left side
- Get back up
- Push-up position plank
- Get back up
- Down on your back
- Get back up

Completing all five series totals twenty-five reps of going up and down—and the body will be hot and sweating. It's a fine warm-up, and it also seems to improve movement. As the movements are restricted (hands on knees), the client needs to come up with new strategies to get back up and down.

For more of a challenge, try these variations:

- Right hand on right knee AND left hand on left knee
- Both hands clasped behind neck
- Putting your hands in your back pockets

Throughout all of this movement, most people, as they tire, will become more and more efficient. When they move to one foot in the lunge position, they will stack their knees vertically over their feet. They will begin to roll and use momentum to continue the movement. Generally, as they tire, most people will do "less."

The movements will become more beautiful as the person simplifies them.

Moreover, it will begin to look like the get-up.

The Get-Up

When in doubt, I pull John Jesse's classic book, *Wrestling Physical Conditioning Encyclopedia* (printed in 1974), off my shelf. Jesse collected the history and wisdom of every strength, conditioning and wrestling coach and compiled it into a rare book that covers all the bases of strength training.

The first lesson one learns when reading Jesse is humility. In case you think YOU invented something, flip through the pages to find:

Swings
Sandbags
Circuit training (including mixing bodyweight work with barbells)
Rehab, prehab, tendon and ligament work
And, many, many more ideas involving equipment, movement and training
Oh…and the get-up

On page 154, we meet Otto Arco. He was the model for many of Rodin's sculptures and we remember him for his skill in one particular exercise:

Arco, at a bodyweight of 138 pounds, could do a one hand get-up with 175 pounds. The get-up was his "secret" to all around body strength, body power and body composition. Arco wrote this in his book, *How to Learn Muscle Control*:

> The main purpose of muscle control is self-mastery. Muscle control involves far more than the mere ability to make the muscles contract. It teaches you to relax, which is sometimes even more important than contraction. It gives you a selective control, and therefore the ability to single out those muscles necessary to the work to be done, and only those muscles; leaving the antagonistic, or non-helpful, muscles relaxed.
>
> That makes a saving of energy in two ways; since it enables you to put all your energy into stimulating the needed muscles, and relieves those muscles of the interference of needlessly flexed antagonistic muscles. Muscle control, which leads to body control, is a great factor for success in all competitive sports.

Arco, over a century ago, singled out the core and keys to the Hardstyle system: "selective control." This is the ability to turn to stone when necessary and to relax...when necessary! It is the secret behind Bruce Lee's one-inch punch and the ability to hit a golf ball far. We find the get-up in Jesse's chapter 13, "All Around Strength and General Power Exercises," where we also discover the ballistic exercises like the swing, the jerk and what we would now call "snatches" in the kettlebell world.

Arco maintained a honed physique that he modeled well into his sixties by focusing on an understanding of muscle-control. While the swing and goblet squat will illuminate the role of flicking the switch of hard/tight and fast/loose, the get-up will demand something best summarized by Jesse (155):

> The athlete, in projecting his total body strength in competition, must mold the strength of localized areas into a total coordinated body effort.

The get-up, sometimes called the Turkish get-up was named after the great tradition of Turkish wrestlers using this move as an entrance test. It has enjoyed a rebirth in the new millennium due to the efforts of members of the RKC. At its simplest, the get-up is simply getting up off the floor with a load and returning back down. It can be done to exacting measures with fourteen or more separate steps up and fourteen or more back down. Somewhere in the middle is how we will teach the get-up.

Although the true benefits are "a total coordinated body effort", when you observe the get-up, you find that many isolation movements are present, too:

- Basic rolling
- Press
- Hinge
- Lunge
- Loaded carry (waiter walk)

We also find the "four knots". The hips and shoulders must be both tight enough and loose enough to roll, slide and adapt through the positions as we move from the ground to standing. Both shoulders are engaged during the full movement at a variety of angles and loading parameters. One needs to be tight and loose throughout as we flow through the positions.

The get-up teaches the ability to remain stiff and tense through movement. When discussing reps for the get-up, I always err on the side of fewer. There are two reasons:

1. Safety is part of performance.
2. Trashing doesn't help tuning.

The first point is the key to the RKC Code of Conduct. Don't trip over a kettlebell haphazardly left on the floor. Don't let go of a swing and hit someone in the face with a kettlebell. Don't go out of your way to be stupid just to become (in)famous on the internet.

Those are all tenants of the "safety is part of performance" idea. With the get-up, a kettlebell is held directly above your skull. The kettlebell will win in a collision, so don't drop it on your head.

More to the point, the get-up teaches total body coordination and total body strength. Like the Olympic lifts—the barbell snatch and barbell clean and jerk—it takes a level of focus to perform a get-up correctly. A single heavy get-up reflects the training base of perhaps months or years to get the movement "right." Like the Olympic lifts, one doesn't see the months of training and preparation that allow one to perform—and, yes, perform is the right word—a heavy get-up.

I keep the reps low to insure concentration, focus and optimal performance. As an Olympic lifting coach, I rarely get over ten reps in either lift with good lifters. With the get-up, I have found that few people can maintain the high levels of mental and physical coordination beyond about ten reps, too.

The second point is hard for many of our hard-charging brothers and sisters to understand: getting trashed is something a college freshman or someone who really doesn't understand training does. I wouldn't be surprised to see someone online doing Tabata get-ups some day (twenty seconds of get-up, ten seconds rest for four minutes) or some kind of "get-ups to failure."

This kind of nonsense is an issue in the fitness industry. Sadly, it is what most people "hear" when we say the phrase "training session".

Even though I want to make you move better and move more, most people's ears tell them that I want you to puke in a bucket and lay in a sweaty mess on the floor.

No!

The get-up is all about tuning the body. The words "tune" and "tone" come from the same root. When we train people, we should be trying to tune them up. If you sit too much, stretching the hip flexor family and strengthening the glutes will do much more together.

When someone struggles in a get-up or cheats a position a bit, it tells us that something is going on today. I use the get-up and variations of it to access what is going on with a person that day. An unusual hitch in movement or a lack of mobility here or there can be addressed instantly if we see the get-up as a tuning exercise rather than a trashing movement.

Speed can mask problems. The get-up highlights weak links and poor linkage. My old training partner, John Price, used to always remind me, "An athlete is only as good as the weakest link." The get-up is a different movement after a trip over ten time zones. The get-up is a different movement the day after an American football game.

But, a few minutes of intelligent corrective work, and tuning the body, allows us to get back into the game.

Stu McGill, the famous Canadian back specialist, offers trainers and coaches a challenge for every workout and program: after the exercises and rep scheme, write a column to explain why each exercise and rep is included.

When it is not included in a workout, we should ask why the get-up is NOT there.

Performing the Get-Up

Before we begin, let's talk about loading the get-up. Generally, I don't like loading the get-up until the trainee can move through the positions without thinking "what do I do next?" There are three simple tools to use in the beginning.

Naked

This simply means "without anything," so don't get your hopes up. Naked get-ups might be one of the best warm ups for general training that I know. Some argue that five minutes of free movement back and forth on both sides without load is great for a warm up period. Oddly, more than a few people have noted that this exercise is "the poor man's chiropractor" as the movement tends to get things popping and snapping into place.

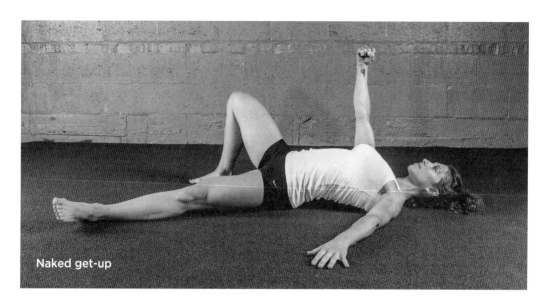
Naked get-up

SHOE (OR SOMETHING FLAT AND LIGHT) ON THE UP FIST

This is a standard for teaching the movement. The loaded arm must point to the zenith throughout the whole movement—and a light load on the fist (THE FIST, not the palm!!!!) insures this basic standard. No one has ever been injured by the falling training shoe.

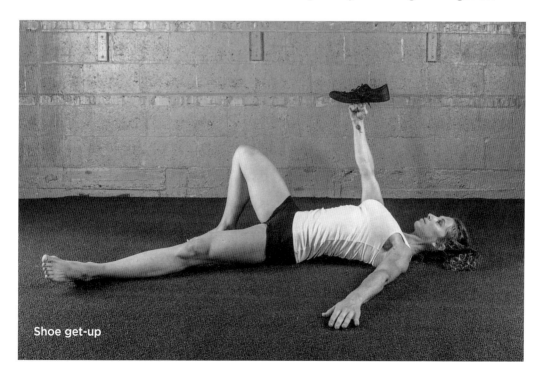
Shoe get-up

A PLASTIC CUP HALF-FILLED WITH WATER

This is the champion for teaching mental focus and keeping the loaded arm at the zenith. Again, the cup is on the fist. This tool teaches the same lessons as the other methods (naked and shoe), but it includes a little punishment for lack of focus. Getting wet seems to teach better than a lot of words, and listening improves during the corrections.

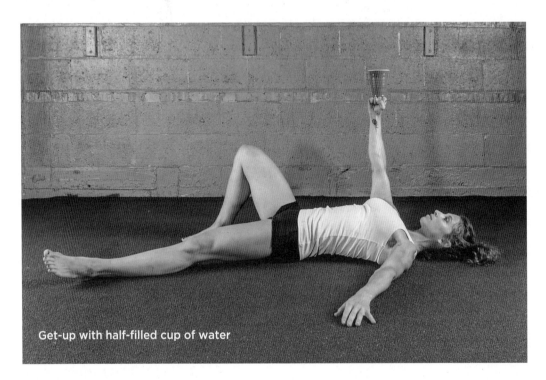

Get-up with half-filled cup of water

I used to teach a class of female high school students and this drill did more to teach concentration and focus than all the lectures, demonstrations, and explanations. A little dousing goes a long way.

How to Get-Up

1. The set up: think 45 degrees and vertical lines

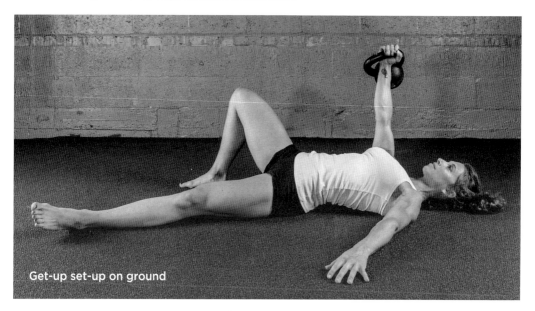

Get-up set-up on ground

2. Roll to side: cross the mid-line and roll up to the elbow

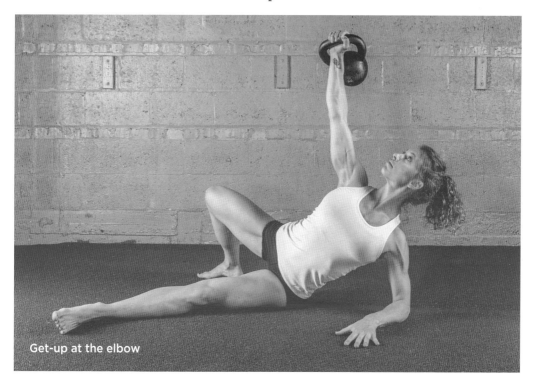

Get-up at the elbow

3. Tall sit

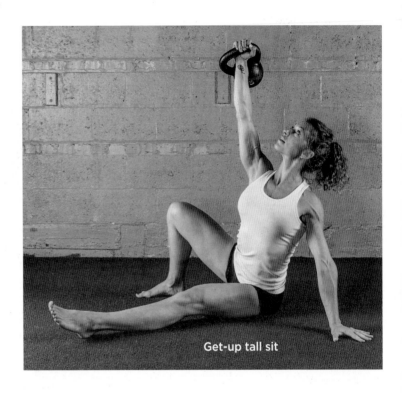

Get-up tall sit

4. Low sweep into kneeling windmill

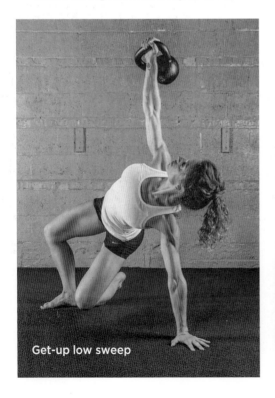

Get-up low sweep

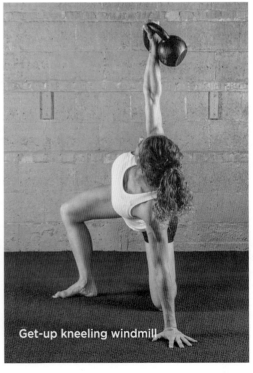

Get-up kneeling windmill

5. Lunge to standing

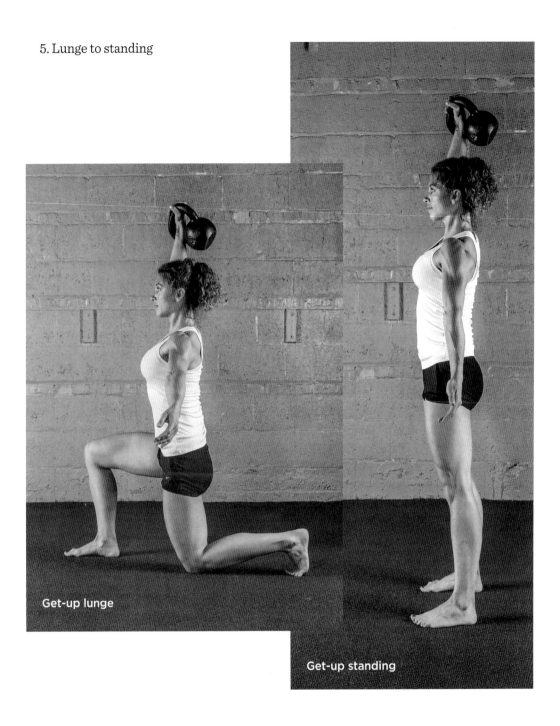

Get-up lunge

Get-up standing

6. Go back down (reverse the order)

7. Change sides

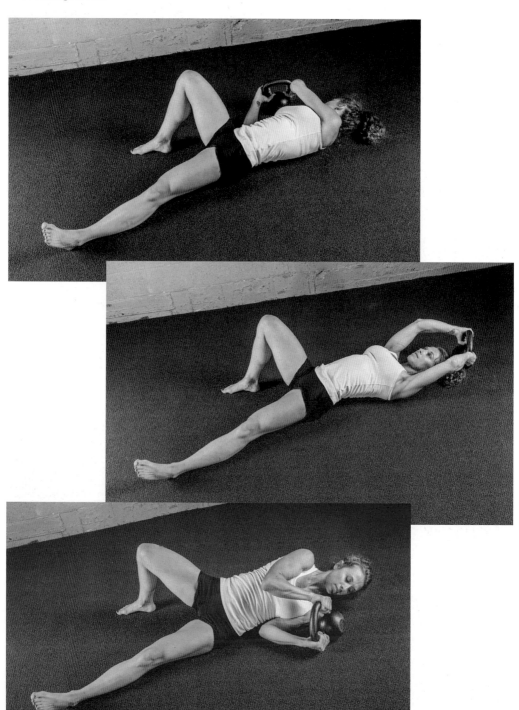

Get-Up Drills

If the exercise was called the roll-up rather than the get-up, I think a lot of problems would disappear. Many people—especially on those horrific internet videos—try to turn the get-up into the crunch-up and disaster ensues. I have a few drills that we practice as part of our regular training that will do wonders for most people.

Rolling 45s

Start on the back, with elbows down at 45 degrees, and legs off at 45s, too. On each rep, be sure the head comes back to the ground. Do not use the neck as the core. Using the elbow as a "wedge," roll up to the elbow position. Check the position of both shoulders, and that both are packed. Roll back to neutral, then roll up to the other side.

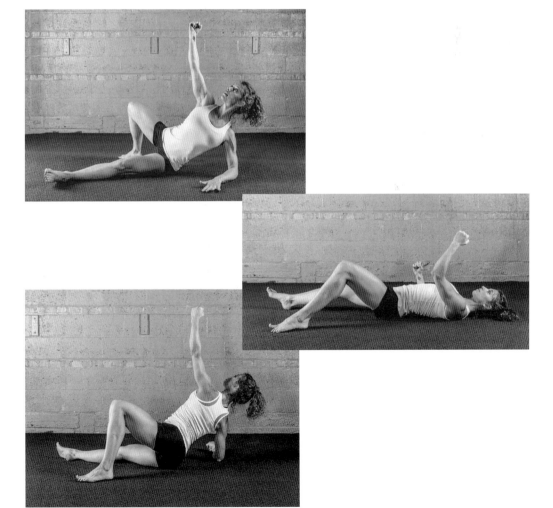

Rolling 45s to the T

Same as the previous drill, but come all the way up to the tall sit position. Be sure the loaded hand is at the zenith and not just flopping around. Roll back to neutral, then roll up to the other side.

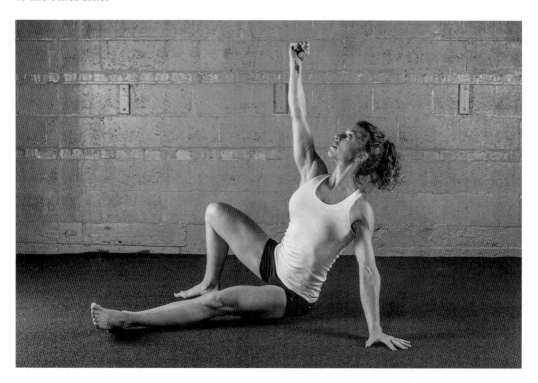

SINGLE KETTLEBELL CARRIES

For many, the get-up's main benefit, shoulder mobility, stability and strength, has been lost due to injuries and "life." The get-up teaches full body linkage, but it might be hard to discover this with jacked up shoulders.

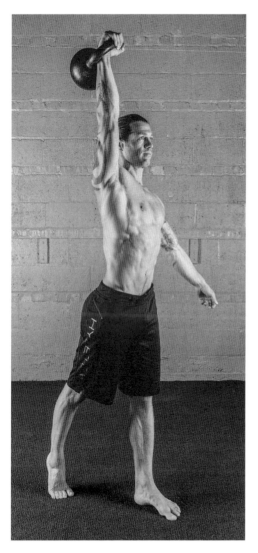

WAITER'S WALK

The weight is held with a straight arm overhead like a European waiter in a café. This is usually the lightest of the carries and does wonders for shoulders.

These variations will either provide more work capacity or serve as a regression for really rough shoulder issues:

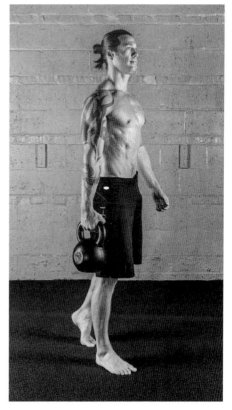

SUITCASE WALK

Grab the weight in one hand like a suitcase and walk. The obliques on the other side of the body will want to have a discussion with you the next day.

Rack Walk

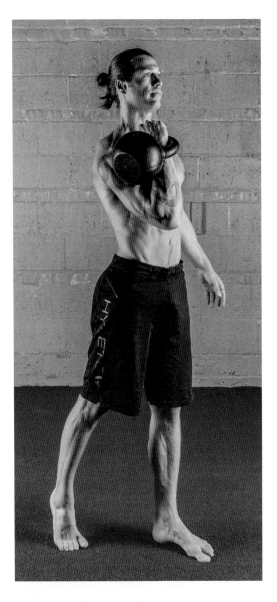

Hold the kettlebell in the racked position, which is the weight on the chest, like a clean. This is a fairly remedial move but it can teach an athlete about how the abs work.

After doing a fair amount of swings and goblet squats, the next way to build up work capacity is to do loaded carries.

Loaded carries also demand integrity. Integrity means remaining in one piece. Moral integrity is being the same person in all situations. In exercise, we don't want to be Frankenstein's monster, a collection of parts. Loaded carries teach integrity under load and movement. Even if you don't want to be a world champion, the following drill has value for everybody.

Gray Cook taught us a wonderful drill that we call the Cook Drill at my gym. (Generally, men can use the 20kg and women the 10kg on the first try.)

Now, begin walking with the weight held fully extended above the head in the waiter walk position. As you continue, wait until you feel like you are losing integrity. Then, shift the weight to the rack. Hold this position until you feel that same loss of integrity. Then, shift to the suitcase carry position.

When you start to lose the integrity in the suitcase position, shift hands and follow the same progression: waiter to rack to suitcase.

Why should we do this drill? Well, for one thing, it exposes our issues. Maybe it is flexibility, the way your spine moves, or something else. I struggle with the rack position because I tend to try to "muscle it" rather than support it. So, let's wake up and train my rhomboids then try it again!

Is it your alignment? Is it your posture? Is it mobility, flexibility, or stability? Is it simply a lack of work capacity? Let's find out: pick up the weight and move for 12-15 minutes! This will give you an insight into your "integrity under load."

Moreover, this drill seems to highlight and improve the issues we may have discovered during the get-up.

Vertical Bird Dog

My brother-in-law, Craig, went to a personal trainer. He had an awful experience. That night, he called me to explain what happened. Simply:

"He wouldn't listen."

No matter what Craig or his wife, Marci, tried to tell the trainer, he rejected it and stayed on his broken record of "more sessions and more supplements."

It's a good reminder for all of us. When someone tells us "this hurts," what is our response? Do you roll your eyes? Do you mentally ping an offensive slur? Honestly, I have done both, but Craig reminds me (and you) that the client and athlete should come first.

Recently, someone said they didn't do bird dogs because "they bother my knees." I looked at the concrete floor and thought (for once!): "You know, a pad would work here."

But, it didn't, and bird dogs still hurt this person's knees. And with that, I tried to fix it. The fix completely changed the way I coach balance, rotary stability, and training the "core."

It's so simple that I am afraid to give it away too soon. Simply, though, I call these "vertical bird dogs." That's right, you do bird dogs while standing up.

In addition, the vertical bird dog family of exercises addresses a big issue. One of the gaps with bird dogs is the lack of load. Now, we can move our hands and legs in circles, squares and then pump the elbows to the knees to challenge stability, but people tend to compensate quickly.

True, many people have experimented with ankle and wrist weights, but the stress on the joints seems to make this even more painful than bare knees on a cold concrete floor.

The load issue is solved by holding a kettlebell—which shouldn't come as a surprise to anyone. Let's look at the Vertical Bird Dog.

I use a series of simple terms to keep clarity in the weight room. Whenever doing an exercise on the knees (half kneeling), we always include these:

LKD: Left Knee Down
RKD: Right Knee Down

For the vertical bird dog, add these:

LFD: Left Foot Down
RKD: Right Foot Down

If you've coached groups long enough, you will have noticed that when you teach the group, your "right" is often the group's left. So, to keep the sequence on track, I recommend ALWAYS doing the left side first and the right side second. Feel free to do the opposite, but stick with one pattern. Our vertical bird dog series will just be discussed LFD (left foot down).

To begin, have everyone stand on one foot. In my book, *Can You Go?*, I note that this is my first assessment. If someone can NOT stand on one foot for ten seconds, I ask them to see a Medical Doctor before we can continue training. I work with several people who have failed this test, and in every case there is a cause. Personally, as I dealt with a necrotic hip joint, I couldn't hold the ten seconds even with my "good" leg. There was something wrong with me and I needed a medical intervention.

So, we all stand on one foot. Stop the drill and move on after about thirty seconds.

From there, we add Taylor Lewis's "Stumble Drill." Maffetone, to remind us, notes that 28,000 Americans die each year from fall and fall related injuries. For years, I taught rolling, tumbling and break-falls to deal with this statistic. But, Taylor had a better idea, teaching people to deal with the stumble. The moment I heard it, I wondered how I could miss something so obvious.

The drill is simple: take your right hand and touch the shoelaces of your left foot. Let the right foot swing up, and then I generally recommend pushing the heel of the right foot straight back, hard.

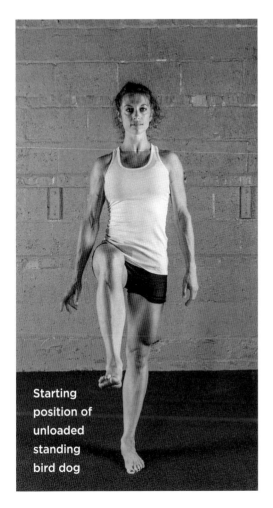

Starting position of unloaded standing bird dog

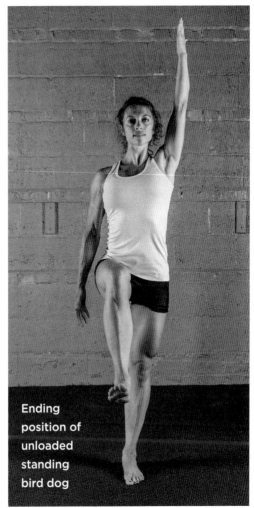

Ending position of unloaded standing bird dog

This can be a hamstring stretch, a deadlift assistance exercise or a test for "gluteal amnesia." Many people tell me that the day after this drill their butt cheeks feel like they marched up a mountain. If you have been ignoring properly training your glutes, you might feel a lot the day after doing this simple drill. In addition, we are practicing "not falling," by catching ourselves before we need to break a fall.

After this, grab your kettlebell. I recommend men start with 20kg and women begin with a 12kg kettlebell. Throughout the drill, keep the kettlebell in the suitcase carry position ONLY.

In the beginning, marching in place with high knees is great practice for the rest of the family of vertical bird dog drills. Marching in place with a kettlebell in the suitcase carry position is also an excellent loaded carry that can complement any training situation with limited space (like large groups).

Mixed with swings, goblet squats and push-ups, marching in place with a kettlebell in the suitcase carry position might be a "perfect" group training sequence.

Now, let's discuss the vertical bird dog family...

LFD WITH THE KETTLEBELL IN THE LEFT HAND

This variation will be relatively easy since the weight is countered by the body mass in this position. Bring the right knee up to at least a 90-degree angle. Feel free to pull it higher.

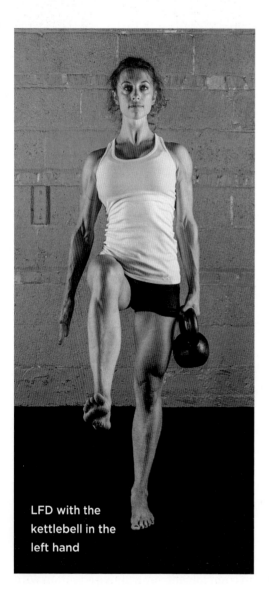

LFD with the kettlebell in the left hand

Switch hands.

LFD WITH THE KETTLEBELL IN THE RIGHT HAND

Now, the kettlebell and body mass are on the same side, so balance will be compromised. The wiggling will completely awaken the entire core of the body. Many report odd soreness the next day in areas like the lats and obliques as the muscles try to adjust and compensate for the demands of balance.

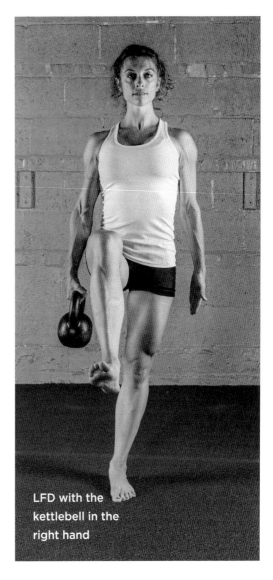

LFD with the kettlebell in the right hand

Now for the fun part: Vertical Bird Dogs

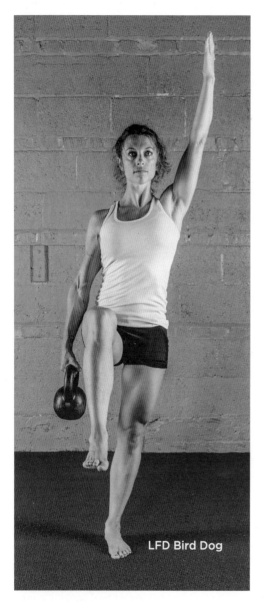

LFD Bird Dog

LFD Bird Dog

With the kettlebell in the left hand, extend the right hand to its zenith. Really drive the middle finger (insert standard joke: important for driving in Utah) towards the stars. The right knee should come up to 90 degrees. Now you are in the traditional bird dog position, except that you are standing up.

LFD Single Side Bird Dog

Switch the kettlebell to the right hand. Now, things get difficult. With the left hand extended straight up to its zenith, the body mass and kettlebell load will pull hard to the right. The left side will need to actively squeeze, release and assess the ongoing struggle to remain upright. If you can hold the stance for a while, the core work is amazing.

One hears the word "activating" a lot recently in the fitness industry and the vertical bird dog family certainly teaches how to activate the whole family of stabilizers (which is essentially every muscle).

Now, simply do the series with the right foot down (RFD).

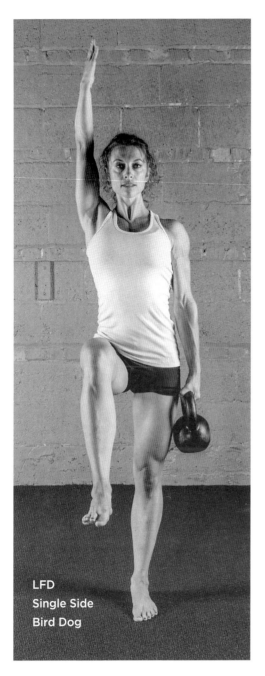

LFD
Single Side
Bird Dog

This series can certainly be practiced daily. One interesting thing: when I jumped up to my 28kg kettlebell (the first kettlebell I ever got, my "Old Blue," my favorite bell), the amount of work necessary to do each drill LEAPED up. So, yes, just like standard training with any lift, the vertical bird dog follows the laws of progressive resistance exercise.

Traditional bird dogs have been a standard in my gym and will remain so. But, "listening" to the issue of hard floors, got me thinking in a direction that I feel will benefit every trainee from the elite athlete to the nice grandpa next door.

You must listen, if you want to be an elite trainer and coach.

Assessment

I have a master list of things I teach young coaches. When I first sit down with them, they tend to want to know the "secrets." I'm sure there are secrets to everything, but in strength training and coaching sports, secrets are as transparent as "buy low, sell high." The secrets are fairly obvious: fundamentals—the basics—are the core and foundation of everything.

I wish I could make it sexier, but the mastery of the basics leads to mastery.

I walk these young enthusiastic coaches through a Ten Commandments of sorts. There are no "shalts" or "shalt nots," but they all carry a fair weight of truth.

Number one is simply constant assessment. The role of the coach, mentor and teacher is to constantly assess and see if we are continuing to go in our intended direction. As with a sail-powered ship, we might need to tack about quite a bit, but we still know where we are heading.

The full list, if you're are interested, is here:

1. Constant assessment.
2. Constant upgrading.
3. Ignore perfect.
4. This isn't Moral Theology—there are no "good" or "bad" exercises or training systems.
5. Everything works!
6. Achieving a goal versus success.
7. After the peak is the cliff.
8. Self-discipline is a finite resource.
9. Fundamentals trump everything else.
10. Take a moment to appreciate those who went before you.

There are many tools to choose from today when discussing assessment. I make a living coaching Track and Field, and the assessment in that sport is simple:

Did you throw farther?
Did you jump higher or farther?
Did you run faster?

If the answer is yes, then we have finished the process of assessment!

Most people won't fit under the banner of athletic performance, so we need some tools to assess them, too. Recently, Doctor Stu McGill noted that just watching a person get down and up from the floor can be a moment for assessment. He asks two simple questions:

Does the person move well?
Are they fit for the task?

Now, the task can be anything...from simply going to the toilet by oneself or finishing an Ironman. I made a simple chart from Stu's insight to help my people understand this first and basic method of assessment:

Simple Assessment From Dr. Stu McGill	Fit for the task(s)	NOT fit for the task(s)
Moves well.	Play ball!	More "conditioning." Needs to get in "shape."
Does NOT move well.	Move regressions, corrections and movement prep.	Progressions, corrections, and appropriats conditioning.

If a person is NOT fit and does NOT move well, take your time teaching movement with any regressions that seem appropriate. I would err on the side of improving movement first.

If the person does NOT move well, but seems fit for the task, our training would be movement-based with the hope of long-term injury reduction and a "balanced" approach to fitness.

If the person moves well, but is NOT fit, then the answer is easy—get in shape, whatever that means for the task. This was most often the case we used to find "back in the day," the person did chores, walked a lot, rode bicycles for fun and played games. To get ready for the task, we just needed to focus a bit on the sport or skill.

Finally, if the person moves well and is fit for the task, then "get in there!" Play Ball! Go out and conquer.

This is obviously a very simple way of looking at clients, but it masks a wonderful truth: many of us can instantly see issues with poor movement and poor movement patterns.

Proper movement is where we begin to reshape our clients—most of the time. Yes, they will want to get sweaty and out of breath, but most of them need to learn to hinge, squat and roll a bit first.

The HKC and Assessment

With the coming of the internet, the fitness industry changed radically. I mention this a lot—back when I first started to train, the monthly magazines (for most of us it was *Strength and Health*) showed up in the mailbox and we often found a new idea or two to try out.

The upside of a monthly magazine is that those one or two new ideas had 28 to 31 days to be tried, tested—and then usually abandoned. But often, something would actually work and this insight would become part of everyone's training. I used to enjoy the articles that combined Olympic lifting and powerlifting (along with intelligent flexibility work) in a program. I learned early that mixing grinds and ballistics took a bit of thinking, but progress was far better when somehow doing both at the same time.

Today, I opened my browser to find ads about a diet that would teach us how to use "tasty carbs" to lean out. The next link touted the benefits of low carbohydrate diets and fat loss. It's a rare day where I am not offered a one-time low-cost opportunity to buy a fourteen, thirty or ninety-day program that will morph me into the best shape of my life.

I always ask, "The best shape of my life for what?" I used to bulk up to 273 pounds then lean out to compete at 242 pounds (110 kilo class). I have thrown the discus really far, but at the same time I had to catch my breath walking up a flight of stairs. I was "in shape" to do the task, the goal, I had chosen years before in a classroom in high school as part of an English assignment.

And, that is the issue: "In shape for what?" I'm as guilty as anyone for listing challenges and getting some excitement going. The 100-rep challenge, picking one global movement and doing 100 singles with it, as well as the various deadlift, farmers walk, and squat challenges, have always been fun. Well, "fun" is an interesting word... But, if you are not competing in a sport, challenges have great value.

We discover that you are in shape for a challenge! This has value, but these kinds of things often don't open the door to further training improvement.

Assessments are great and I use the FMS, our own gym's 1-2-3-4 Assessment, plus all of the various smaller tools, tips and gadgets to assess where you are and what you need to address in the future.

But sometimes, you realize that a test or assessment no longer really assesses or tests, it has become a challenge. I used to use two basic tests: one-minute of push-ups, and max pull-ups.

I had a student do 111 push-ups in one minute. He was a short-armed wrestler and counting the reps was an issue at that speed. How could he top that score? I honestly have no idea. And, what would be the value to work to get 112 for an athlete who wrestles?

I had another student do 66 pull-ups in a row. Again, he was born to do pull-ups, but even if you got half his score (33 for the math impaired), you are still amazing.

I discovered that most of my tests were becoming marathon races or specialty events where genetics would trump actual training. There is still value in a bodyweight press and double bodyweight deadlift, of course. But as I worked through the assessment process, I added some built-in buffers to make counting reps more reasonable and the impact of proper training clearer.

I also began to realize that the Hardstyle Kettlebell Three (swing, goblet squat and get-up), plus my old standards the push-up and pull-up, were an amazing toolkit for testing and assessing.

I would like to share these in the order that I began adding them to our system.

THE 30-SECOND HANG PULL-UP

Gray Cook first opened my eyes to hanging and pull-ups. It was a simple idea: if you want to test someone for max pull-ups, test their hang (for time) from both the straight arm position and the flexed hang position, before you test their max reps.

Many people lack the grip endurance to deal with max pull-ups! Gray argues that the best way to increase the pull-up, as well as save the elbows, is to practice and increase the hang time from the straight and bent arm positions.

We took this one step farther for testing and assessment: each pull-up begins with a 30 second hang.

So, "One" is a 30-second hang, then a pull-up.

"Two" is a 30-second hang, then a pull-up—then ANOTHER 30-second hang and a pull-up.

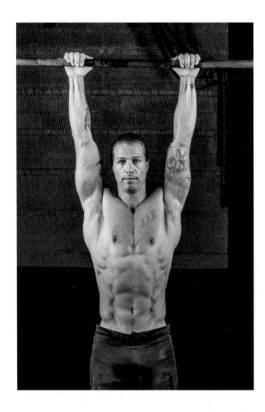 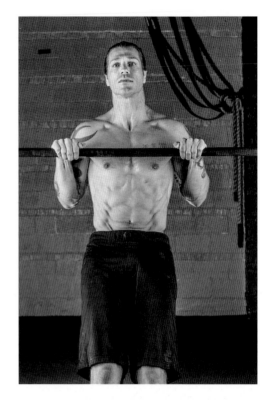

Completing two reps in the pull-up test takes just over a minute. If you can do four in this method, then you are doing just fine. The ease of counting total reps, as well as judging the reps is so much easier than the traditional Q and A after every rep: Did the chin get over? Were the arms straight? I know that the arms will be straight for the bulk of the time on the reps with this method.

No one has yet reported completing six reps, though one person claims a score of a five. In full candor, I don't care what the best can do, but getting two or three is pretty solid.

One great insight from many men is that the "gap" is shoulder mobility/flexibility. It's not grip strength, but "jacked up" joints that hold people back on this test. Getting stronger might not be the right answer to passing the test, it might be mobility and corrective work.

The Six-Minute Squat

The pull-up test led us to the goblet squat test. I'm sure you can do this with any squat, but the goblet squat gives an interesting challenge to your "anaconda" muscles, the muscles that you use to squeeze things ("I love you!") and the "cobra" muscles—the ones that pop up in your back that make you look you have a hood. Some call these "trapezius muscles," but I didn't go to medical school.

Sit in the bottom of the goblet squat for thirty seconds. Grunt and stand up. Then pull yourself back into the bottom position. Stand up at the 30 and 60 second mark. Generally, this test lasts about three to six minutes.

Finish standing and park your kettlebell like a professional. I am always shocked how sore my biceps, ab wall, and odd parts of my outer back feel for the next two days. Yes, I work those muscles, but the time under load is the issue here. Moreover, we learn a lot of interesting things about our hip and back mobility as we hold the deep squat for the workout.

This is a simple test/workout to describe, but it's oddly difficult to do.

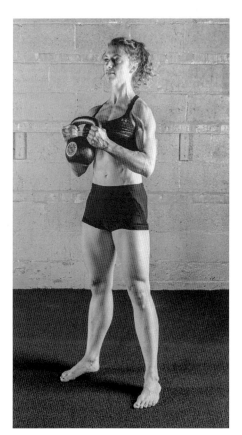

A typical man would use the 24kg kettlebell, and ladies can choose the 16kg or 12kg. Five minutes (ten times standing up) should be a nice line in the sand for you to walk over. I have done this several times for six minutes and I am not sure there is much value going beyond that time.

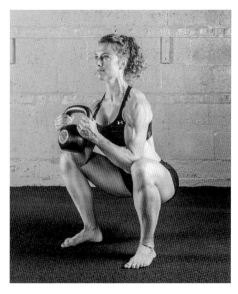

The Proper Push-Up Test

The push-up test has been an issue for us to measure. Did the arms straighten out? Did the chest touch the floor? Is the plank maintained?

Proper push-ups eliminated these problems. We got the idea from Gym Jones: basically, when you go to the bottom, lay your chest on the floor and stick your hands out to a "T" position. Return your hands to their previous position, then press up. That's a proper push-up.

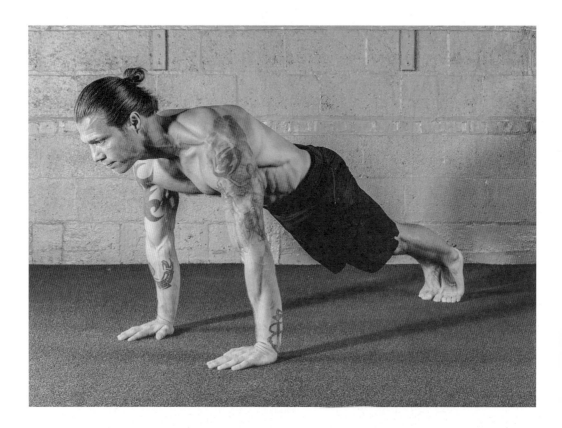

This idea has made testing and assessing much easier: there are no more questions about touching the floor or issues with saggy bodies. Moreover, counting is much easier as this cuts the volume in half for most cases. A one-minute proper push-up test will be flying at 30 reps.

Strive to complete at least 20 proper push-ups in this test. Note how the descent will remain much more controlled for most people. I am sure a few will decide to free fall to increase their reps, but this form of self-CPR has little value to the general fitness or performance enthusiast.

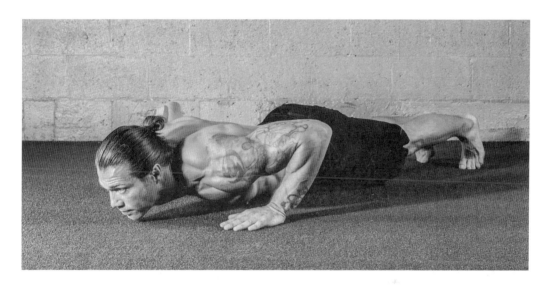

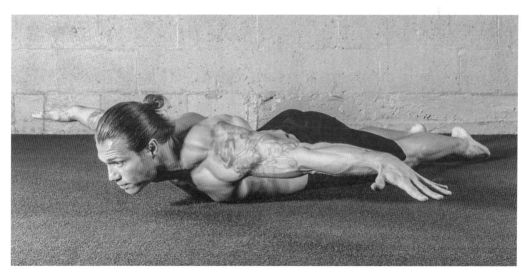

The Five-Minute Get-Up

I first heard about "slow motion" competition from Dan Millman of the *Peaceful Warrior* series. His idea for true mastery was to do your event as slowly as possible. Without an implement, practicing the track and field throwing events as slowly as possible lends some insights into orbit and transitions that can be unexamined at normal performance speed and tempo.

RKC Team Leader Chris White mentioned that he did "Five-Minute Get-Ups" at our RKC in San Jose and I wanted to slap myself for missing such a simple idea. Rather than crash through a bunch of reps, glide and hold each position while doing a full body "check in" to see if everything is aligned and appropriate.

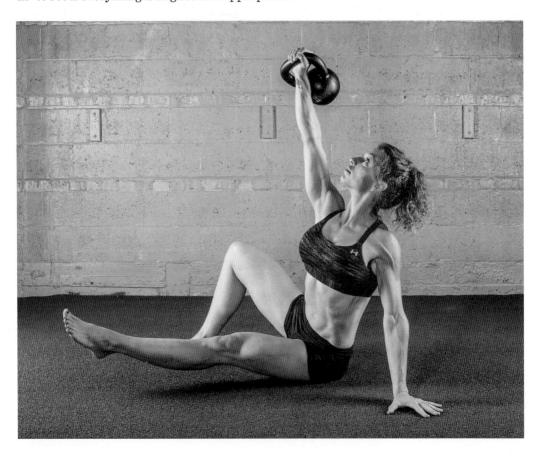

At first, try adding leg or foot lifts at every logical stopping point. I find simply picking up each foot highlights issues with positioning or compensations. Parts of the get-up are hinges, squats, rolls and lunges, and picking up a foot can sometimes illuminate why we seem to thrash or cheat through this position.

I would imagine the ultimate get-up would be to continuously move through the entire five minutes. For mortals like me, a naked get-up done very slowly with an attempt at seamlessness would be the first line of assessment.

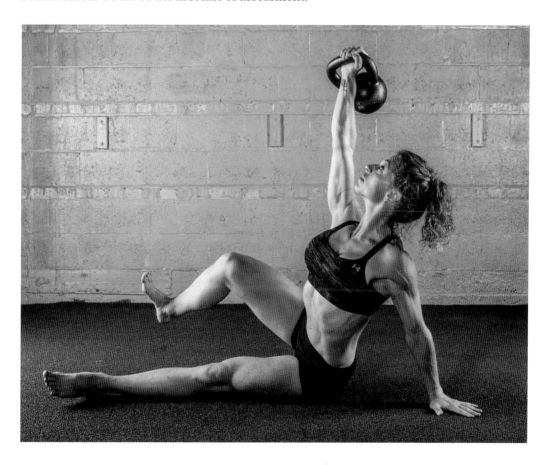

Extra Credit: Two-Minute RKC Hip Flexor Stretch

Along the same lines as the five-minute get-up, consider doing the RKC Hip Flexor Stretch for extended periods. Try two minutes per side at first. Like in a good yoga class, you will find that spending more time in the position allows a deeper release of the stretch. That might sound more like voodoo, but extending the time in this stretch is pure gold.

Fifty Swings

During our first 10,000 Swing Challenge, we discovered that our grips were not what we thought in terms of strength and endurance.

The original rep scheme:

- A set of ten swings
- One rep of a strength movement
- A set of fifteen swings
- Two reps of a strength movement
- A set of twenty-five swings
- Three reps of a strength movement
- A set of fifty swings

Repeat four more times for a total of 500 swings.

Most of us discovered an interesting fact when using an appropriate kettlebell—our grips gave way after thirty reps. Swing technique begins to degrade with grip issues and you should put the kettlebell down.

So, the "test" is to do fifty swings with your RKC Snatch Test kettlebell and maintain a proper grip!

As with all of our simple tests in the HKC family, this one is easy to write and read...but hard to do!

Adding the pull-up and push-up tests to the HKC Three gives you five interesting test/assessments to push you further along the path. The upside of each of these tests is that none of them truly have a finish line. I can still imagine someone bragging on Facebook about having the slowest get-up ever. These tests will each highlight some basic issues in not only strength or power but in areas like mobility and flexibility.

My search continues for tests, assessments and evaluations that will continue to challenge people to strive for better, not "more."

HKC™

Programming the HKC

The problem with programming is simple: the word "program" is sitting right there to start off the word "programming." And, programs are the problem.

It's not an unusual week when someone emails me asking for a "program." It's not unlike a patient calling a doctor to ask for medicine. There seems to be a logical question as a follow up:

"Um, for what?"

There are a million programs out there in books, magazines and the internet. Most bodybuilding magazines will provide about a dozen conflicting and complicated programs guaranteed to terrorize your triceps, pound your pectorals, and blitz your biceps.

There are programs for fat loss, muscle gain, and athletic peaking. I imagine they are all good and work perfectly as written. Sadly, few people ever follow a program for more than a few workouts.

Few of us ever actually FINISH programs. So, we end up with dozens of starts and misfires when it comes to doing programs and we miss the big picture.

Jim Wendler (inventor of the 5/3/1 program) recently wrote this about his mentor:

> Towards the end of my senior year, I finally asked Darren why he never spoke to me during my first year in the weight room. And it was this lesson that I have taken with me in all areas of my life. His answer:
>
> "Because you hadn't earned it. I've written hundreds of programs and helped so many kids and teachers with their training—and almost all of them quit after the first week. I had to see if you were going to stick with it. I had to see if you were serious. I'm not going to waste my time or my energy."

For most of us, programs are two to twelve weeks of following a structured workout that usually builds up to a peak week and a max. It is nice if there are easy days, maybe some deloading weeks, and some logical means of increasing load or volume...or both.

But, most people quit them after the first week!

Programming is the big picture. Armed with an understanding of programming, one can occasionally shift into these structured two to twelve-week training blocks to address issues and fix problems.

There are three keys to understanding programming. These come from the HKC manual, but are expanded in both the RKC and RKC-II certification curriculum. The keys are:

- Continuity
- Waving the Loads
- Specialized Variety

Understanding these three terms and applying them appropriately to any training model, piece of equipment or situation will allow you to progress towards any body composition or athletic performance goal.

Continuity

The secret to success in life is usually pretty simple. Woody Allen once noted, "90 percent of success is simply showing up." The same is true in fitness and performance: pack in enough workouts and training sessions over time and good things will happen.

Good things happen when we focus on continuity in training.

Pat Flynn summarized training like this:

- Train consistently for progress.
- Add variety for plateaus.
- Add randomness for fun.

Continuity can be summed up as "Train consistently for progress." And, there is nothing new here. Most of us know the story of Milo.

Milo was a wrestler and multi-time Olympic champion in the original Games. His father-in-law was Pythagoras, who made life easier with his idea that "The sum of the areas of the two squares on the legs (a and b) equals the area of the square on the hypotenuse (c)." We are also told that Milo consumed twenty pounds of meat, twenty pounds of bread and eighteen pints of wine daily. But, that is not why we remember Milo. It was his idea to pick up a bull.

The story goes that each day he would walk out to the pasture and pick up a certain calf. The next day, he would repeat this until the bull was full grown. Milo is the father of progressive resistance exercise and it's his fault that many people think success in strength training happens in a straight line. I have joked many times with new lifters that if you bench one hundred pounds today and only add ten pounds a week, about a year from now you will bench over 600 pounds. It sure works on paper.

At some level, we all know Milo was right. During and after World War II, Dr. Thomas DeLorme and Dr. Arthur Watkins were working with polio patients and injured soldiers. In 1945, DeLorme wrote a paper, "Restoration of muscle power by heavy-resistance exercises," published in the *Journal of Bone and Joint Surgery*.

In 300 cases, he found "splendid response in muscle hypertrophy and power, together with symptomatic relief," by following this method of 7-10 sets of 10 reps per set for a total of 70-100 repetitions each workout. The weight would start off light for the first set and then get progressively heavier until a 10RM load was achieved. Over time, the workouts changed in terms of volume.

By 1948 and 1951, the authors noted:

> "Further experience has shown this figure to be too high and that in most cases a total of 20 to 30 repetitions is far more satisfactory. Fewer repetitions permit exercise with heavier muscle loads, thereby yielding greater and more rapid muscle hypertrophy."

A series of articles and books followed where they recommend 3 sets of 10 reps using a progressively heavier weight in the following manner:

Set #1 - 50% of 10 repetition maximum
Set #2 - 75% of 10 repetition maximum
Set #3 - 100% of 10 repetition maximum

In this scheme, only the last set is performed to the limit. The first two sets can be considered warm-ups. In their 1951 book, *Progressive Resistance Exercise*, DeLorme and Watkins state, "By advocating three sets of exercise of 10 repetitions per set, the likelihood that other combinations might be just as effective is not overlooked... Incredible as it may seem, many athletes have developed great power and yet have never employed more than five repetitions in a single exercise."

I love that last line.

Furthermore, at about the same time, Vladimir Janda, the physician and physical therapist, began his great insights into tonic and phasic muscles and his various "crossed syndromes." It is also important to note is that he was a victim of that terrible disease of the last century, polio. Janda's concluded that stretching (loosening) one muscle and strengthening its opposite would promote better structural integrity than just attacking one side of the equation.

Janda also taught us that certain muscles tighten when we get ill, injured or aged. The "tonic" muscles—pectorals, biceps, hip flexors and hamstrings are key for most people. Other muscles (phasics) weaken when we get ill, injured or aged and include the glutes, deltoids, triceps and abs.

The Hardstyle Kettlebell Three work miracles to counteract both the stretching of tonics and weakening of phasics.

Continuity of training embraces the idea that we need progression. Reasonable progression. Solid training programming looks at building the load, the reps, and the sets up over time.

But, we also have to be realistic. I have had to sit down with many proud fathers and explain to them that their belief in their child's linear progression does NOT hold up under the lens of common sense.

Billy benched 100 pounds as a 14-year-old. Dad projects his improvement to be about ten pounds a month. So, next year, Billy will bench 220 pounds, which seems doable. The next year, at age 16, Dad sees him at 340 in the bench press, and I begin to wrinkle my nose. At 17, Bill (he is now grown up), should be benching 460. You can see where this is heading.

To get better in any field or quality of life, we must remind ourselves of my college coach's key to success, "Little and often over the long haul." Ralph Maughan knew athletics and life: "little and often over the long haul" should be one's mantra for most of life's work.

- Continuity is showing up.
- Continuity is training consistently for progress.
- Continuity is progressively adding volume or load.
- Continuity is being reasonable about expectations.

Once you embrace continuity, you can now shape your workouts by "waving the load."

WAVING THE LOAD

To understand *Waving the Load*, you need to consider three terms:

- Volume
- Intensity
- Density

Volume is a math problem. If using just a single kettlebell, this is a pretty simple operation:

Add up all the reps in your workout(s) and compare them to other workouts.

Volume is the tough one for me. Ten total reps with a 48kg kettlebell in the press is the same "volume" as twenty reps with a 24kg kettlebell. Determining which workout is harder (48kg for 10 versus 24kg for 20) has been the subject of discussion in lifting circles for generations.

There is a method for figuring out an appropriate "volume to load" ratio for Olympic lifters and I applaud it. The issues come with adapting it to other lifting forms.

Carl Miller introduced an interesting concept to Olympic lifters in the 1970s. It was called "K Value" and it is based on a formula. Olympic lifting is judged by tallying the best of two lifts, the snatch and the clean and jerk. So, the contest total will be the sum in the discussion.

To calculate the K Value (I thought of saying "simply," then caught myself), we first need this information:

1. The total load of training.
2. The total number of repetitions.
3. The "total" made at the competition (the sum of the best snatch and clean and jerk).

The total load of training is determined by the total number of repetitions done with each weight lifted in major exercises. So, the athlete needs to multiply each weight lifted by the number of reps completed.

Then, we take the total number of reps (number two) and divide it by the total load—so, load divided by reps. We then multiply THAT number by 100 and divide that number by the "total" made at the competition (number three).

At the time, Bulgarian Olympic lifters were averaging scores around 40, while most Americans were in the lower 30s. It demonstrated that the Bulgarians were really pushing load with their volume...a tough thing to do!

Considering that a lifter might have 700-1000 lifts in a training cycle, I think you get a sense of the issue with K Value—the MATH! My coach, Dick Notmeyer, had me do the math equation one time and I learned to stop asking so many questions!

Of the three (volume, intensity and density), it's the hardest to convince people that "more is not better" with volume. Yes, I am a champion of things like "The 10,000 Swing Challenge," but crappy swing technique will do far more damage than good.

My advice for volume:

1. Always keep an eye on load when increasing volume. There is a great value in doing more reps with a lighter load, for example, practicing the 100-rep snatch test. Light loads with volume have a "tonic" effect, in the old use of the word…it makes you feel better. But, enough is enough.

2. You should only rarely increase volume more than 50% of your current levels. One of the issues with the 10,000 Swing Challenge is that many people go from 75 to 500 swings in their first workout. Yes, it is doable, but the hands and grip take a beating that might have been saved by easing into the reps.

3. If you are getting ready for performance, cut volume and focus on other qualities.

4. Generally, when volume goes up, intensity (next discussion) tends to go down. It is true that the answer to the classic question, "Which is better: heavy weights or high reps?' is "Both!" But as mere mortals, we can only handle so much.

We now need to discuss intensity to truly understand volume.

INTENSITY

I'm not sure if fitness and training has any words more confusing than intensity. Yes, intensity is the amount of weight used in training. Yes, it is how close you are to failing or missing the lifts.

The devil is in the details.

When Arthur Jones sold his Nautilus machines through the massive advertisements in *Scholastic Coach* magazine, he redefined intensity. It became the rep one failed while using a machine with perfect form (on a machine). Some define intensity by how much vomit ends up in a bucket. Some define intensity by the percentage of maximum lift.

The last one is good, but fraught with issues. I have a different set of terms for the word "max."

From "Sorta Max" to "Max Max Max"

First, let's look at three highly scientific terms that I use on a daily basis:

- Sorta Max
- Max Max
- Max Max Max

The Sorta Max

Most people have a "Sorta Max." A Sorta Max is a concept I thought up a while ago after hearing people tell me their "max" in various lifts. Sorta Max is that heavy lift you do in the gym and call it a day. And, I must say this, hats off to you, you deserve it. That's great, nothing wrong with it. It's the "heavy for today" max, if you will.

Many of us will occasionally have a good day and nail a big lift, or in some cases, just have a great performance. That's where most people hail their "max" numbers.

The Max Max

Max Max is the next step. That's that top end lift that maybe you spent the better part of a few months building up to with some kind of organized program. For the record, that's exactly what my best bench press reflects.

John Price and I decided at least three times that both of us needed to bench press 405—four big plates per side—and focused on the bench for two workouts a week. It was a very simple workout and we just tried to push our reps up. It always worked.

If I had ever spent more than a month working on the bench, I'm sure I could have done more. But, for me, 405 is/was my Max Max. A few weeks of training focused on one lift and I made a good number.

In my opinion, the Max Max is the most underappreciated measure in sports and training. It's simply what you can do with some effort. If all your Max Max numbers are at a good level for your goals and interests, I can practically promise you that you have achieved a solid level in your chosen field. Maybe not the best, but you're good.

THE MAX MAX MAX

Now, it should be obvious where Max Max Max is heading. This is a number that takes a lot of commitment and a lot of time to achieve. You'll probably need to do it in competition. All my top lifts are done in competition. Why? Well, there's usually a story.

Why a 628 deadlift? Because after I pulled 606, a bunch of other guys missed, and then one or two went up and made a big show of missing something a bit heavier. So, I wanted to make sure there was no question—I took the next poundage up (628) and made it.

So, Max Max Max might be a lifetime achievement that you either planned for decades or, like me, you simply stumbled around long enough to do something "max-worthy." And that's the issue.

When novices plot out a "Max," we need to have the follow up question. "What do you mean by max?" I have been to many RKC certifications and talked with someone who had a "max" kettlebell in a lift. But, a day of coaching, demonstrating and practice often leads to a new "max."

Any and all training based on the old max numbers certainly had value, but was probably under-loaded for the period.

There is nothing wrong with that!

There is great value in playing with variations of load and intensity.

Low volume/low intensity: these training sessions are where we practice skills and actively recover. These might be the most underappreciated sessions.

Medium volume/medium intensity: these sessions should probably be three out of your five workouts. You get the work done and leave feeling better than when you arrived. These sessions won't be posted on social media, but they are the ones that lead to growth and change.

High volume/high intensity: these are the sessions we brag about later. Generally, we take our time building up to these sessions and need some easy days afterwards. An example would be the five ladder and five rung day of the "Rite of Passage". For this workout, I did 75 clean and presses with my left hand, another 75 with my right hand, and 75 pull ups. After that, I did a ten-minute snatch test! That is a lot of volume. In addition, I only had my 28kg kettlebell at the time, so the intensity sneaked up very high.

High volume/low intensity: as noted, these workouts, used appropriately, can be part of the building process leading to a peak or improved performance.

Low volume/high intensity: these are the sessions designed to push through a new max or limit lift. Like high volume/low intensity, these workouts are crucial to building up to a peak.

Good programming uses all five methods. Generally, week in and week out, focus on the medium volume/medium intensity method for most of the workouts. Mix in perhaps a low volume/high intensity day with a low volume/low intensity recovery day. One can train for a long time with a program like this.

Plan the "low/low" days after any kind of "high/high" day. In a group of five workouts, I generally suggest the following:

- Three medium/medium days.
- One "high" day (volume or intensity).
- One low/low recovery, tonic and practice session.

If you take on weeks of "high" on either side of volume or intensity, be sure to plan some sessions afterwards for the opposite with low/low mixed in.

For example, after the twenty days of 500 swings (The 10,000 Swing Challenge), we shift over to three days a week of mobility/tonic workouts focusing on, at most, 75-150 swings total while mixing in stretching, rolling, and mobility work. There might be one "heavier" session during the week focusing on heavier grinds.

DENSITY

Density is getting the work done in less time. With volume, the tool is the calculator, or an abacus if you are like me. With load, the tool is simply the heaviest kettlebell you move.

With density, the extra tool is the clock.

More work. Less time.

There are two ways to attack density. The first and probably the most obvious way is to get through a workout noting the start and end time. Then, the next time you do this same workout, you finish it faster.

That's it.

For many, the problem will quickly become obvious: racing through a workout often leads to poor technique. You MUST have quality control. Putting a kettlebell down "like a professional" while panting and heaving is a matter of discipline. If you can't insure proper technique, proper performance and proper safety, stop and slow down.

It's a race against yourself that you will want to repeat again sometime soon. Don't lose your future trying to win today.

The other methods are work to rest ratios. Let's look at the most common:

1:1

This can be difficult. Generally, this is 30 seconds on, then 30 seconds rest/active recovery. If the exercise is kettlebell swings, you will swing for 30 seconds and then do "Fast-Loose" drills for 30 seconds.

For many, less time is an issue. 15 seconds on and 15 seconds off often requires a level of skill and precision that many people simply don't have…yet.

With a partner, this method is known as "I go/you go."

1:2

This is the rest period we use in "cohorts." Cohorts are three person groups training together. The rest period increases by the additional of another person. "I go/you go/you go." With exercises that need more recovery—for example double kettlebell front squats—this will give the body time to recover for another set.

1:3

This is how I learned to lift. We worked in groups of four and everyone took their turn. This is very good for grinds, Olympic lifts and powerlifts in group and team settings.

TABATA

This is twenty seconds of movement followed by ten seconds of rest for four minutes. I think this works with squats and, honestly, nothing else. It is a workout that leaves people in a pool of sweat with their dog trying to call 9-1-1 without thumbs! This popular workout interval has been so bastardized that its original vision has been lost. Use it with common sense.

Density training probably makes the best kind of kettlebell workouts. The same workload in less time works well with kettlebell ballistics and complex workouts like double kettlebell clean and push jerks. I would suggest using heavier kettlebells or changing the workout, after doing five workouts where the same load is done in less and less time.

As good as density can be, enough is enough.

Specialized Variety

Specialized variety can be summed up in two ways:

- "Same, but different"
- "Fun"

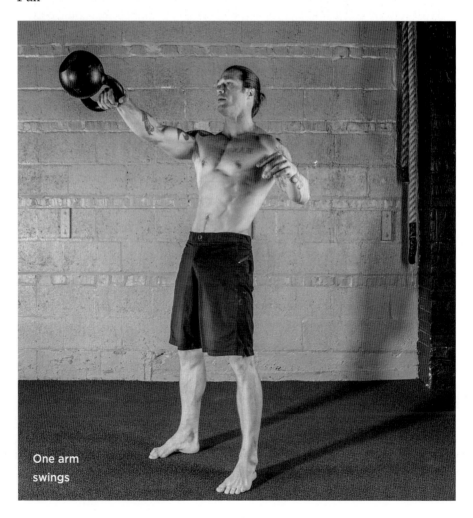

One arm swings

Pat Flynn's other two principles apply here: "add variety for plateaus" and "randomness for fun." Most people who have trained for a while know the basics.

With barbells, switch out front squats for back squats or incline bench press for bench press. When Dick Notmeyer had me do back squats after four years (!!!) of just front squats, I felt like a new man. It was the same thing, basically, but it was actually fun.

If you are bored with two hand swings, shift to one arm swings, or double kettlebell swings, or dead stop swings or...

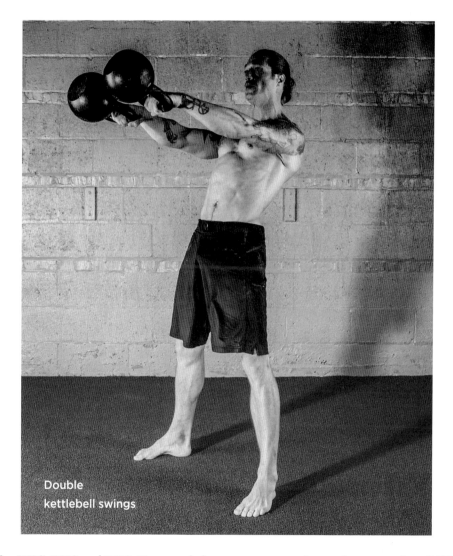

Double kettlebell swings

The HKC, RKC and RKC-II manuals have many pages devoted to examples of different moves and variations for every movement.

But...

It is not just fun and an attempt to deal with boredom. Biology teaches us that we adapt to stress and stimulus. We learn to accommodate (the law of accommodation) and get better and better at things with less and less effort.

For body composition training—basically fat loss for most—I suggest that we need "inefficient exercise." Simply, if you are really good at something, you probably won't stress your fat reserves doing that movement.

If you were a former collegiate swimmer and put on fifty pounds of fat, swimming—especially now that you are more buoyant—might not be a good fat loss option for you as you are too talented (and floaty) to get much from the laps.

Let me explain it this way: I have a neighbor who has a tricked-out racing bike, aerodynamic helmet, and, yes, a white spandex racing suit. White. As in "almost see through."

He also has a magnificent beer belly. His problem is simply that his bike rolls effortlessly around our streets and he doesn't work very hard to get in his miles. My bike, a cruiser, weighs about seventy pounds and has a beer bottle opener built in.

It's a struggle to pedal my bike up a small incline. Riding one hundred miles on this big tire, beer-holding bike would be an effort!

If you can't swim well, struggling back and forth in a pool is a great workout. If you float and glide, it might not be much of a day.

Inefficient exercise drives fat loss.

So, when you get too good at certain moves, you drive the reps up, but perhaps not the energy usage. One thing we noticed in the 10,000 Swing Challenge is that towards the end, we have figured out ways to save energy. We have learned to "cheat" the swing.

We have become "efficient."

So, we need to change the exercise with specialized variety. We will still do the movement, but with a different variation.

SIMPLIFIED PROGRAMMING

With an understanding of volume, intensity and specialized variety, we can now move into the basics of programming. I always start with the fundamental human movements as my guide to appropriate programming:

- Push
- Pull
- Hinge
- Squat
- Loaded Carries
- Everything Else

"Everything else" can be tumbling, lunges, monkey bars, correctives—everything else. Often, these movements—especially anything done on the floor—have great value beyond fitness and performance and into the realm of survival. If you need to crawl to safety, save your joints in a fall, or climb out of harm's way, these skills will trump a big bicep curl.

Loaded carries and hinges build athletes. The loaded carry family trains the body to work as one piece and provides the stability Stu McGill calls "stone." When you hinge into someone and turn to stone, that person is going to be hit hard. These two movements are the key to athletic performance.

The push, pull and squat are both hypertrophy and power/strength movements. I have one rule: the volume of push, pull and squat numbers must be exactly the same each week. When you send me a "program," there are two things I look for:

1. Gaps. Which fundamental human movement are you NOT doing?
2. The balance of the push, pull and squat numbers.

Often, I find these volume numbers over a week for American lifters:

Push: 237 reps
Pull: 135 reps
Squat: 15 reps

This is why I love Delorme's concept of "basically" 15 to 30 reps of an exercise. The classic workouts reflect this:

3 sets of 8
5 sets of 5 (Reg Park workout)
5 sets of 3
3 sets of 10 (as seen above)

Doing the same rep and set scheme for the push, pull and squat insures that there will generally be balance in the body. Many American males need to add more pulls to balance the years of over pressing and pushing.

So, some programming "rules" are emerging:

1. Do all of the fundamental human movements.
2. Push, pull and squat rep numbers must have the same totals.
3. Use the hinge and loaded carry families to improve athletic qualities and work capacity.
4. Include enough of "everything else" to keep the client functioning and safe.

To see how I do this, let me include this example. For an explanation of the extra movements, go to my YouTube page, dj84123.

I call the sixth set of movements in my training "everything else" to sound a bit more professional. It's not unlike putting my name on my polo shirt: it doesn't really add any credence to what I say or do, but it looks like I know what I am doing.

MONDAY

- Naked get-ups
- 15 Swings, 5 goblet squats, march in place
- Stoney stretch (RKD)
- 15 Swings, 4 goblet squats, march in place
- Windmill stick "look right"
- 15 Swings, 3 goblet squats, march in place
- Naked get-ups
- 15 Swings, 2 goblet squats, march in place
- Stoney stretch (LKD)
- 15 Swings, 1 goblet squat, march in place
- Windmill stick "look left"

Subtotal:
- Hinge: 75
- Squat: 15

Do Two Rounds:
- 25 Swing variation (hip thrusts)
- 5 Double kettlebell front squats
- 15 Swings
- Mini-band walk
- Farmer walk

- Pull-ups: 3-2-2-2-1
- One-arm kettlebell press: 1-1-1-1-1

Do Two Rounds:
- T x 25
- Ab Wheel x 5
- 25 Swing Variation (Hip Thrusts)
- 10 Swings plus 5/4/3/2/1/ Goblet Squats

Total:
- Push: 5
- Pull: 60
- Hinge: 230
- Squat: 40
- Loaded carry variations: 2
- Sixth movements: 4

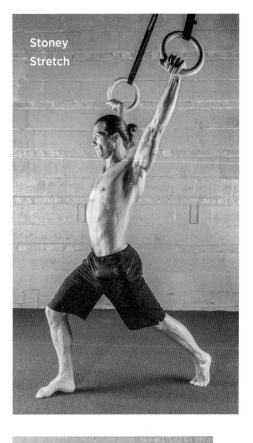

Stoney Stretch

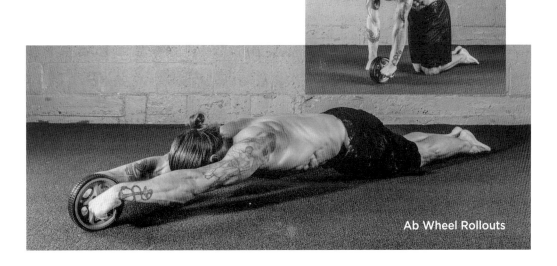

Ab Wheel Rollouts

THE HARDSTYLE KETTLEBELL CHALLENGE

TUESDAY

- Naked get-ups
- Hip thrusts x 10, 15 swings, 5 goblet squats, march in place
- Stoney stretch (RKD)
- Hip thrusts x 10, 15 swings, 4 goblet squats, march in place
- Windmill stick "look right"
- Hip thrusts x 10, 15 swings, 3 goblet squats, march in place
- Naked get-ups
- Hip thrusts x 10, 15 swings, 2 goblet squats, march in place
- Stoney stretch (LKD)
- Hip thrusts x 10, 15 swings, 1 goblet squat, march in place
- Windmill stick "look left"

Subtotal:
- Hinge: 125
- Squat: 15

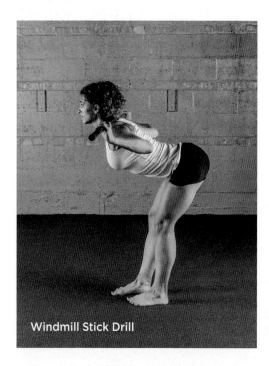
Windmill Stick Drill

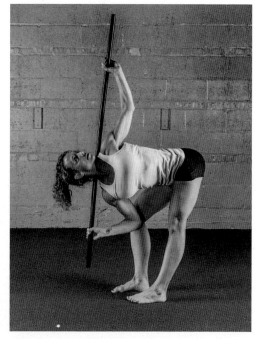

Do Three Rounds:
- 8 x T-Y-I rows
- 5 Ab wheel roll-outs
- Hip Flexor Stretch R/L

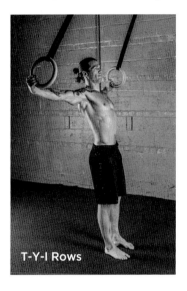
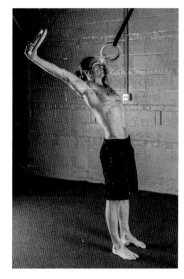
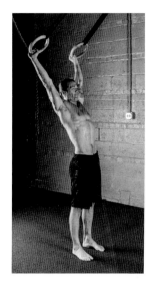

- Pull-ups: 3-3-2-2-1
- One-arm kettlebell press: 2-1-1-1-1

Do Three Rounds:
- RING biceps curl x 15
- RING triceps extension x 15
- Bear crawl-bear hug with Judy x 2

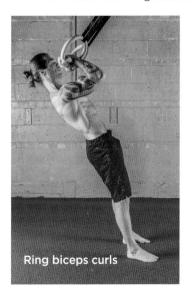
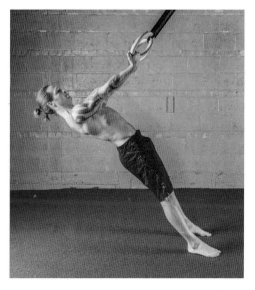

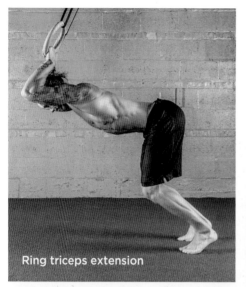

Ring triceps extension

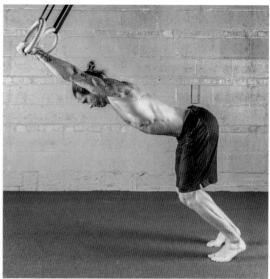

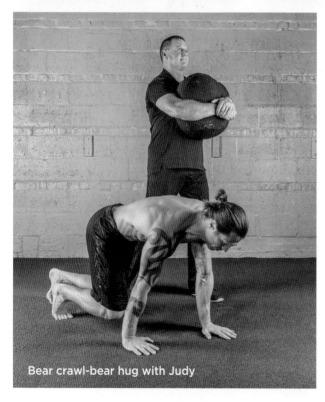

Bear crawl-bear hug with Judy

Total:
- Push: 6 (45 extensions)
- Pull: 83
- Hinge: 125
- Squat: 15
- Loaded carry variations: 2
- Sixth movements: 4

Thursday
- Naked get-ups
- Hip thrusts x 10, 15 swings, 5 goblet squats, march in place
- Stoney stretch (RKD)
- Hip thrusts x 10, 15 swings, 4 goblet squats, march in place
- Windmill stick "look right"
- Hip thrusts x 10, 15 swings, 3 goblet squats, march in place
- Naked get-ups
- Hip thrusts x 10, 15 swings, 2 goblet squats, march in place
- Stoney stretch (LKD)
- Hip thrusts x 10, 15 swings, 1 goblet squat, march in place
- Windmill stick "look left"

Subtotal:
- Hinge: 125
- Squat: 15

- Pull-ups: 3-3-3-2-1
- One-arm kettlebell press: 2-2-1-1-1

- Double kettlebell press: 2-3-5-10 (Finish all twenty reps before moving on to the hip thrusts. Between sets do rocks, hip flexor stretches and be a general nuisance.)
- Hip thrust x 25
- Goblet squats x 10
- Suitcase carry

Three Total Rounds:
- Round One: Light Double Presses
- Round Two: Heavy Double Presses
- Round Three: Medium Double Press

Total:
- Push: 67
- Pull: 12
- Hinge: 200
- Squat: 45
- Loaded carry variations: 1
- Sixth movements: 4

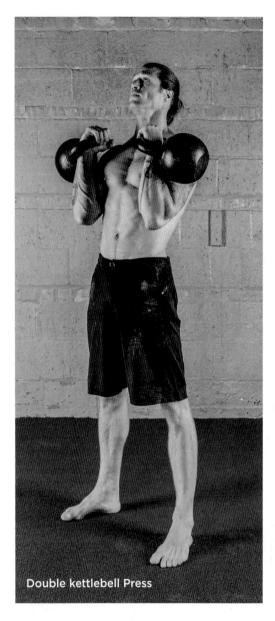

Double kettlebell Press

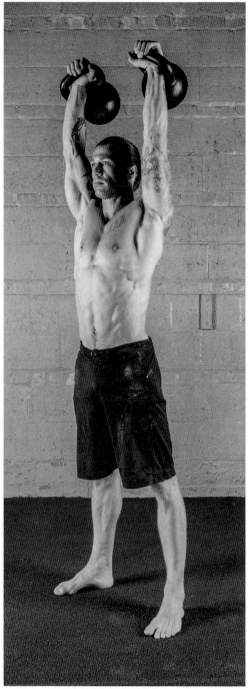

Friday

- Naked get-ups
- 15 Swings, 5 goblet squats, march in place
- Stoney stretch (RKD)
- 15 Swings, 4 goblet squats, march in place
- Windmill stick "look right"
- 15 Swings, 3 goblet squats, march in place
- Naked get-ups
- 15 Swings, 2 goblet squats, march in place
- Stoney stretch (LKD)
- 15 Swings, 1 goblet squat, march in place
- Windmill stick "look left"

Subtotal:
- Hinge: 75
- Squat: 15

- Pull-ups: 1-1-1
- One-arm kettlebell press: 1-1-1

- Mini-band walk with black band
- Double kettlebell front squat x 3
- Waiter walk
- Double kettlebell front squat x 3
- Farmer walk
- Double kettlebell front squat x 3
- Light sandbag carry
- Double kettlebell front squat x 3
- Medium sandbag carry
- Double kettlebell front squat x 3
- Heavy sandbag carry
- Double kettlebell front squat x 3

Do Two Rounds:
- Ring Triceps Extension x 15
- Ring Biceps Curls x 15
- KB French Press x 15
- Barbell Curls x 15

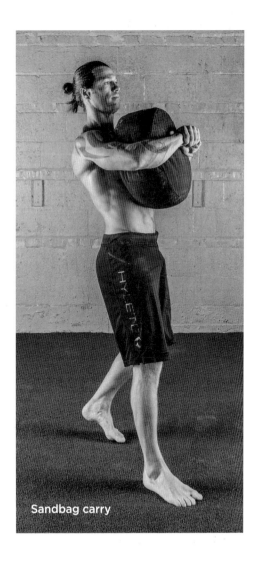
Sandbag carry

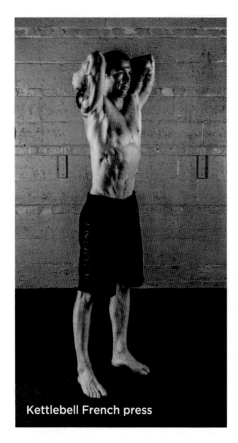
Kettlebell French press

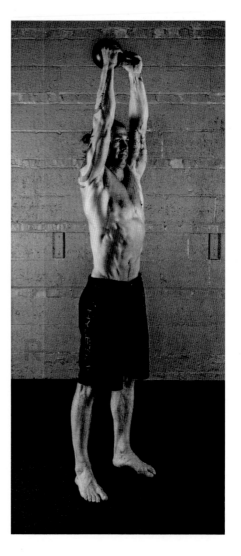

Total:
- Push: 3 (plus 30 extensions)
- Pull: 3
- Hinge: 75
- Squat: 33
- Loaded Carry Variations: 6
- Sixth Movements: 2

Weekly Totals:
- Push: 81 (plus all the extensions)
- Pull: 158
- Hinge: 605
- Squat: 133
- Loaded Carries Variations: 11
- Sixth Movements: 14

This is NOT a template for you to run off and follow! It's advanced preseason training for a football player or thrower. But, this example should give you the planning vision for weekly work.

Please note that this plan includes a lot of pulls. Many of our throwers have long careers and busted up shoulders, so they need more pulls. Our collision sports guys (American football) also have issues with the shoulder area.

I always ask groups, "Raise your hand if you have shoulder problems." Watching the struggle to raise a hand above shoulder height is a pretty good assessment of this big problem.

Training a "normal" person will be much easier, but the ideas behind their training must be discussed first. The word "fractal" comes to mind. A fractal is a never-ending pattern. Fractal patterns are already familiar, since nature is full of them in trees, rivers, coastlines, mountains, clouds, seashells, and hurricanes. A leaf looks like a tree, a small stone looks like a mountain. If done correctly, a training day can look like a career.

Jurassic Park discusses this same insight from another perspective:

> "And that's how things are. A day is like a whole life. You start out doing one thing, but end up doing something else, plan to run an errand, but never get there... And at the end of your life, your whole existence has the same haphazard quality, too. Your whole life has the same shape as a single day." — Michael Crichton

I have a simple model for training most people:

It's life.

Here's a training program based on our movement history:

1. We start off rolling around and crawling.
2. Then, we get up on one knee.
3. Then, we go back down to the ground.
4. We finally rise up and go after it for a while.
5. We stumble and get back up.
6. We stumble again and lay back down.
7. And then we stay down!

This is also a great template for training.

1. Naked get-ups (no weight) and ground-based mobility work.
2. Half-kneeling presses (alternate with both knees down), do a few reps with each hand.
3. Bird dogs.
4. Humane burpee or variation (see below for examples).
5. Mobility movements from six-point position and half-kneeling.
6. Naked get-ups.
7. Easy foam rolling or correctives.

The goal of this session was to "get sweaty" and build some strength. But most importantly, it was designed so you could leave the gym feeling better than when you got there.

This training session can be expanded or contracted as appropriate. For a vision of how to train a typical trainee, try the following monthly template.

Classical Conditioning

A = Light (50%) B = Medium (75%) C = Heavy (100%)

For this program, the weight is based on what you can lift for ten repetitions, not for a single lift. So, it will be a load that you can "sometimes" lift for eight reps and sometimes for twelve, depending on life. Never miss a lift.

Program A – Simple Strength

Getting stronger is the foundation of all fitness goals. Stretching during rest periods keeps the intensity—including heart rate—up. Strive to increase "C" over time.

Push: One-arm press
- A x 10
    Hip flexor stretch L
- B x 5
    Hip flexor stretch R
- C x 10

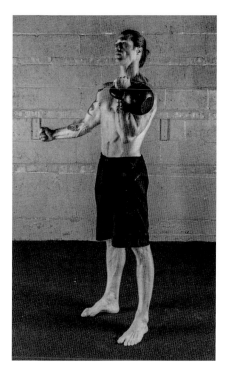

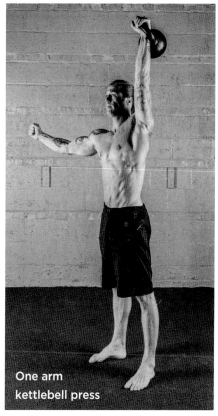

One arm kettlebell press

Pull: One-arm row
- A x 10
    - T-spine mobility work L
- B x 5
    - T-spine mobility work R
- C x 10

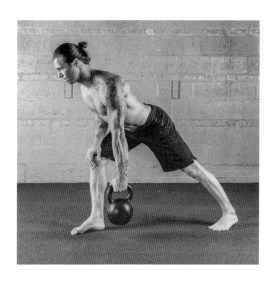

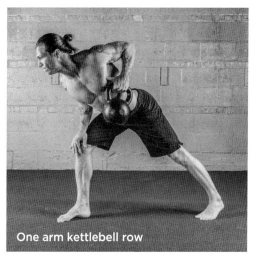

One arm kettlebell row

Hinge: Swings
- A x 30
    Bird dogs
- B x 15
    Bird dogs
- C x 30

Squat: Goblet squat
- A x 10
    Pumps (cobra and downward dog)
- B x 5
    Pumps (cobra and downward dog)
- C x 10

Plank: Push-up plank for two minutes or less

Carry: Farmer or suitcase carry

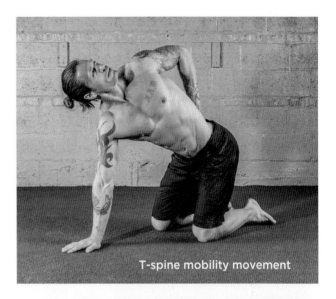

T-spine mobility movement

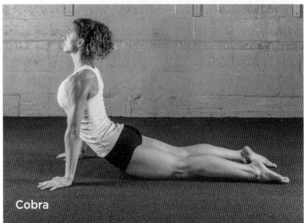

Cobra

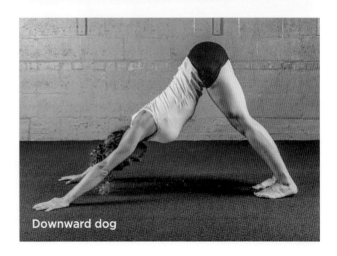

Downward dog

Program B – The Cardio Hit Workout

For the past few years, mixing the dynamic swing with the grinding squat has been an interesting way to increase heart rate. Adding stretches between sets will keep the heart rate high, but will also add some heart rate variability (a good thing). Don't hold the stretches for more than thirty seconds; pop up for another set of swings.

- 15 Swings, 1 goblet squat
    - Hip flexor stretch L
- 15 Swings, 1 goblet squat
    - Hip flexor stretch R
- 15 Swings, 1 goblet squat
    - T-spine mobility work L
- 15 Swings, 1 goblet squat
    - T-spine mobility work R
- 15 Swings, 1 goblet squat
    - Bird dog
- 15 Swings, 1 goblet squat
    - Bird dog
- 15 Swings, 1 goblet squat
    - Pumps (cobra and downward dog)
- 15 Swings, 1 goblet squat
    - Pumps (cobra and downward dog)
- 15 Swings, 1 goblet squat
    - Push-up plank
- 15 Swings, 1 goblet squat
    - Suitcase walk L/R

Program C – Tonic Recharge Workout

This is the workout which should follow a Tabata day. Yes, this is an easy day, but the focus is always on the long-term goal and the journey.

Push: One-arm press
- A x 10
    - Hip flexor stretch L
    - Hip flexor stretch R

Pull: One-arm row
- A x 10
    - T-spine mobility work L
    - T-spine mobility work R

Hinge: Swings
- A x 30
    - Bird dogs
    - Bird dogs

Squat: Goblet squats
- A x 10
    - Pumps (cobra and downward dog)
    - Pumps (cobra and downward dog)

Plank: Push-up plank
- 1:00

Program D – Bi-Monthly Tabata

We only use a ten-second rest, so alert your client to be ready to go again at seven seconds. Please use a Tabata timer, many are available for free on the web.

We go for twenty seconds, rest for ten, and then repeat the sequence another seven times for a total of eight rounds—just four total minutes of working out. Stay focused.

Remember, the rest periods are only ten seconds, be ready to go again at seven seconds. Go after it today.

- Time #1
    - Tabata goblet squats for 4 minutes total
- Time #2
    - Tabata swings for 4 minutes total

Program E – The Mobility Workout

Hold each position for thirty seconds. Participants under thirty years of age are recommended to go through the movements for two circuits (do every movement once, finish the list, repeat). Participants age thirty to fifty, go through the movements for three circuits. Over fifty, complete the circuits at least three times, but strive to do four or five.

- Hip flexor stretch L
- Hip flexor stretch R
- T-spine mobility work L
- T-spine mobility work R
- Bird dog
- Bird dog
- Pumps (cobra and downward dog)
- Pumps (cobra and downward dog)

Progression or Regression— Adjusting the Weight

Bryan Mann from the University of Missouri did an interesting study using the DeLorme and Watkins protocol. The previous workout was based on their training insights using the 10-5-10 on the strength movements. His insight on standardized progression was very helpful, and he proved that the old-school methods still work. Use the following general template to adjust the load for future training sessions.

Based on the number of reps completed for set number three, reduce, maintain or increase as follows:

- **4–5 reps:** Reduce the weight by 5 to 10 pounds next time.
- **6–8 reps:** Maintain the weight or reduce by 5 pounds next time.
- **8–12 reps:** Maintain the weight next time.
- **12–15 reps:** Increase the weight by 5 to 10 pounds next time.
- **15+ reps:** Increase the weight by 10 to 15 pounds next time.

If your client only completes 0–3 reps on the heavy set, you either overshot the weight estimate, or there's something else going on. When the numbers for each of the third sets put the client in different categories (for example, 7, 9, 12, and 15), you may need to make an educated estimate for the next session.

SUN	MON	TUE	WED	THUR	FRI	SAT
Rest	Program A *Simple*	Program E *Mobility*	Program B *Cardio*	Rest	Program A *Simple*	Program D-1 *Goblet Squats*
Rest	Program C *Tonic*	Program E *Mobility*	Program A *Simple*	Rest	Program B *Cardio*	Program C *Simple*
Rest	Program A *Simple*	Program E *Mobility*	Program B *Cardio*	Rest	Program A *Simple*	Program D-2 *Swings*
Rest	Program C *Tonic*	Program E *Mobility*	Program A *Simple*	Rest	Program B *Cardio*	Program C *Simple*

This program ties in well with the volume/intensity recommendations above. Warm ups are not mentioned, but generally I recommend a few minutes of get-ups and basic mobility work. Cool downs would be the same, but opposite: basic mobility work followed by get-ups. Program E, the mobility workout, is a fun day to see how mobility helps "smooth out" the get-up work.

The devil is in the details with programs and programming. I would argue that FLEXIBILITY is the key here. The goal is not touching your toes, but understanding that things change, life happens, and perfection is a tough goal. I strive for "pretty good" when it comes to programs and programming with a hint of "that's not bad" tossed in for luck.

You will adapt and learn and relearn. Billy Graham once said, "If you find the perfect church, by all means join it! Then, it won't be perfect anymore!"

If you find the perfect program, by all means DO IT! Then, it won't be perfect anymore!

General Principles for the "Rest of Us"
Lessons from Elite Athletics

One of the hardest things to understand as a weekend warrior or general fitness enthusiast is that the tools and lessons of elite performance sports have great value and can really point us on the right path. Every so often, the sports networks will highlight an athlete who sleeps in a high-altitude chamber, drinks kale smoothies every few hours and has a two-hour deep tissue massage daily.

That all sounds great, but for most of us, just getting in twenty minutes of exercise a day might be an effort of time management and free will worthy of an epic handed down for twenty generations. Magazines and TV shows love to show the guy using magical herbs and bizarre foods rather than the bulk of the performers who just eat good food.

On the exercise side, it can be worse. You rarely see a commercial with a professional athlete training with a barbell or kettlebell. Almost always, they have bands, straps, computers and cast offs from NASA experiments. It's hype and you should know that by now. Most of us—along with elite athletes—simply need to train and get their workouts in the weight room finished. Then, we build on it.

I have five principles for supporting our training:

1. Train appropriately for goal(s).
2. Train little and often over the long haul.
3. The longer it takes to get in shape, the longer the shape will remain.
4. Warm-ups and cool-downs really do play important roles.
5. Train for volume before intensity.

First, be sure your training matches your goal. If the goal is fat loss and general health, mix a training program with elements of cardio, hypertrophy and mobility. If you want to win a triathlon, it would be nice to know how to swim and bike. If you are an athlete, use your sport to condition yourself for the sport and the weight room to build the qualities of strength, mobility and hypertrophy.

Even weekend warriors quickly learn that you can't make up for five days of commuting and sitting in a desk by going after it for two days every weekend. You must find time for short workouts that will support your weekend plunges. It takes eight to twelve years to build an Olympian. Give yourself a few extra days to support your fitness goals.

Training little and often over the long haul relates to the next point. The longer you take to get in shape, the longer you seem to stay in shape. Six week and ninety-day body transformation programs are fine, and they work well for those who finish, but a six-year approach to conditioning will be a lot better for the medal count. Take your time getting in shape.

I don't think we always need to have a perfect warm-up or take the time to cool down. Sometimes, your name is called and you have to be ready. However, for most of our efforts, a warm up and cool down period will give you a chance to get some work done in the other areas of training: foam rolling, flexibility, discussion of tactics, planning for upcoming trips and competitions and general community building. The warm up and cool down period is often the best time to both plan and reconsider the plan towards your goals.

Finally, most of us need to train with a lot of volume before we light up the intensity. I believe in intervals for runners, peaking for lifters and "crunch time" for team sports. But, you can't do it all the time. Do the work and build a foundation with the lower intensities and build a foundation. Once or twice a year, feel free to "go for it."

Just remember, you might not have the support staff and money to go for it 365 days a year. None of these principles are earth shattering or original, but check them against what you are currently doing. During times of illness, injury, or generally lousy training, circle which of the five principles you ignored and strive to NOT make that mistake again in the future.

From "General" to Specific: One-Kettlebell Workouts

A common request after the HKC is: "Can you give me more workout ideas?" Let's review the minimum effective dose for each movement:

- Swings: 75-250 a day
- Goblet squats: 15-25 a day
- Get-ups: 1-10 each side a day (As RKC Team Leader Chris White reminds us, "Just doing ONE get-up slowly over five minutes is as instructive as anything you can do.")

I think if we add 15-25 push-ups a day, we might have a routine that will provide fitness, longevity, health and performance.

Yet, the devil is in the details.

How much equipment do you have?

Surprisingly often, many people have only ONE kettlebell. Or, we find situations with large groups where clients only have one appropriate kettlebell.

There is a niche in this industry for one kettlebell workouts. I love them. I enjoy driving to a park, meeting with friends, walking a bit with my kettlebell, training, and then having a nice picnic. I keep this tradition alive every weekday morning when people join me to workout at 9:30AM.

I would like to explore the many options we have with one-kettlebell workouts.

Most people want "workouts," but "training sessions" is a better term. We need to spread out our fingers a bit and look at programming. I always talk about programming as the "Four Twos":

- Two Decades
- Two Weeks
- Tomorrow
- Today

I always ask the client or athlete to look twenty years down the line. The checks you write with your body doing "hold my beer and watch this" stunts will be hard to pay twenty years from now. "Just because you can, doesn't mean you should," the best lesson of *Jurassic Park,* is also wise programming guidance.

Two weeks is just about the longest most people will follow a diet or program. I'm actually exaggerating; with diets, it is barely two hours. But, let's look ahead two weeks and circle the issues and problems that will lead to missed workouts or bad choices in food and beverages. Can we deal with this proactively?

Tomorrow is my favorite. I always tell people that "Tomorrow will be the greatest workout of my life. I will destroy all records, leave myself in a sweaty mess, vomit often, and have one near death experience."

Today? Oh, today, I will do the fundamental human movements with appropriate reps, sets and load and strive for mastery of movement.

When tomorrow comes around I tell everyone, "Tomorrow will be the greatest workout of my life. I will destroy all records, leave myself in a sweaty mess, vomit often, and have one near death experience."

Tomorrow never comes!!!

Smart training and smart programming focuses on the big picture of two decades!

To make daily training sessions, let's first look at swing-focused workouts. One quick hint: don't let the press dictate your kettlebell selection, especially with women. Recently, my group traveled the "Rite of Passage". On one heavy workout, one of our females just picked up the 28kg and did five minutes of swings. She didn't notice that what she thought was a 20kg kettlebell was actually a full 8kg heavier.

She realized that she had been using too light a load for swings. She had built up to the 16kg in the "Rite of Passage", but she could easily use more weight for the swings and goblet squats.

These workouts are JUST for two-handed swings, but feel free to adapt them as appropriate. Moreover, as one person told me not long ago, "Just do 30 seconds of swings, 30 seconds of 'Fast-Loose' drills—then try to add minutes when you can."

Simple!

A few years ago, I was asked to write about the 10,000 Swing Challenge. Basically, one sets aside twenty days and adds 500 swings per workout. If you swing four times a week, it takes five weeks; we usually did 500 swings five times a week, so it only took us four weeks. "Yay" for us.

This is the simplest version:

- Swing 10 reps
- One goblet squat
- Swing 15 reps
- Two goblet squats
- Swing 25 reps
- Three goblet squats
- Swing 50 reps

Rest. That is 100 repetitions, so just swim through it for an additional four times—for a total of five giant sets.

An interesting version of the get-up will really get your heart pumping (groundwork seems to oddly increase HR):

- Swing 10 reps
- One get-up, weight in left hand
- Swing 15 reps
- One get-up, weight in right hand
- Swing 25 reps
- Two get-ups, one left and one right
- Swing 50 reps

A small note: I always go left side first when it comes to any one hand, one leg or one foot movement. That way, I never need to remember what to do next. Ignore this at your own peril with large groups.

One could certainly do push-ups, pull-ups or nothing between sets of swings. We found in our fourth 10,000 Swing Challenge that this variation saved our grip with heavier kettlebells:

- 15 Swings
- Goblet squat, get-up, or whatever
- 35 Swings
- Goblet squat, get-up, or whatever

Repeat for an additional nine times for ten total giant sets. This workout allowed us to use heavier kettlebells, and it also doubles the longer rest periods.

Many people will ask about "rest." Since these workouts are focused on density, FINISH the workout, and stop where you need to stop for the first few times. I think that natural rest periods trump programmed rest periods. If a strong man is using a light kettlebell, he may not even need to take a single break.

Rest periods are the ultimate "it depends" situations.

I love combining the swing and push-up. Getting up and down from the floor seems to be as hard as the two movements! I asked my friends to come up with their favorites...and here they are:

WORKOUT OPTION #1
- 20 seconds swings
- Push-ups 6 reps
- 30 seconds rest

Repeat for 15 minutes

* Per workout, increase push-up reps by 1

WORKOUT OPTION #2
At the top of the minute:
- 20 swings, 10 push-ups, rest the remainder of the minute.
- 20 swings, 9 push-ups, rest... and so on down to
- 20 swings, 1 push-up.

If you want to do 15 minutes, start with 20 swings, and 15 push-ups.

Next time do 21 swings each time...

WORKOUT OPTION #3
- 20 Swings
- Gather yourself
- 10 Push-ups

* Note: Instead of time, add sets

WORKOUT OPTION #4

- 20 swings
- 20 push-ups
- 20 swings
- 15 push-ups
- 20 swings
- 10 push-ups
- 20 swings
- 5 push-ups
- 20 swings

Total = 100 swings, 50 push-ups, 0 fluff

WORKOUT OPTION #5

- 20 swings
- 8-10 push-ups
- 30 second plank
- 1 minute various hip stretches

Repeat for 20 minutes

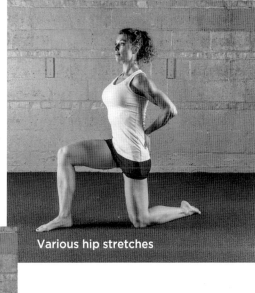

Various hip stretches

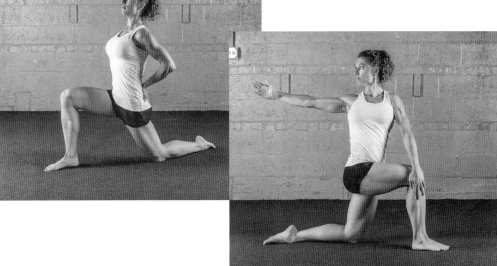

There is a million ways to do these workouts, but these five workouts are a nice little group.

Now, adding the goblet squat turns everything on its head. As we go through the next section, I tend to do things in this order:

- Swing
- Goblet squat
- Push-up

Swings tend to be ten or fifteen reps, goblet squats NEVER more than ten (and usually five reps) and the same for push-ups (never more than ten and usually five).

My favorite variation is "The Humane Burpee." Dan Martin gave it this name and I can't think of a better term. You can certainly make it harder or easier, but just try the basic example first.

Be sure to follow the advice about reps on the goblet squat and push-up: we want the reps to descend as we move through the "Humane Burpee," hence the name "humane."

So, here you go:

- 15 Swings
- 5 Goblet squats
- 5 Push-ups

- 15 Swings
- 4 Goblet squats
- 4 Push-ups

- 15 Swings
- 3 Goblet squats
- 3 Push-ups

- 15 Swings
- 2 Goblet squats
- 2 Push-ups

- 15 Swings
- 1 Goblet squat
- 1 Push-up

That comes out to 75 swings, 15 goblet squats and 15 push-ups. The real exercise seems to be the popping up and down for the push-ups. Most of us don't take any rest at all through the workout, but feel free to stop when you need to rest.

To make it harder, just slide the goblet squats and push-ups reps up to ten. 10-8-8-7-6-5-4-3-2-1 gives you 55 total reps and that is plenty of work for a single day....in many cases, it's too much.

I have three more variations that have value:

I'm not sure why this is called "Slurpees," but it is:

- 10 or 15 Swings
- 5 Goblet squats
- 10 Mountain climbers (every time the left foot hits counts as a rep).

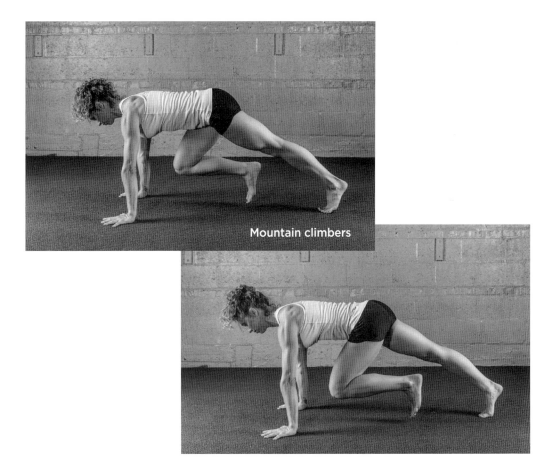

Mountain climbers

Let the goblet squats descend (5-4-3-2-1). That gives you 50-75 swings, 15 goblet squats and a lot of heart pounding.

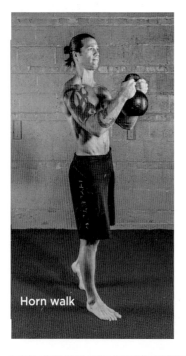

Horn walk

"Hornees" are the first of our loaded carries. A horn walk is simply walking around with the kettlebell on the chest. It keeps the tension high.

- 10 or 15 Swings
- 5 Goblet squats
- Horn walk for an appropriate distance.

Again, let the goblet squats descend (5-4-3-2-1). That gives you 50-75 swings, 15 goblet squats and an interesting feeling in the whole area of muscles that squeeze things together.

"Bearpees" are great for groups:

- 10 or 15 Swings
- 5 Goblet squats
- Bear crawl

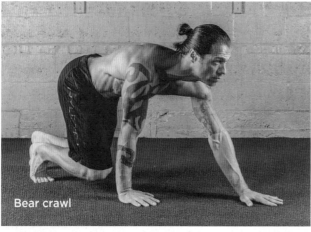

Bear crawl

Again, descend with the goblet squats (5-4-3-2-1). In groups, you can have teams of two people, 60 feet apart and they share the same kettlebell. You will see a lot of racing and the participants will quickly learn that they have underestimated the intensity of crawling.

Once we get moving with horn walks and bear crawls, it is time to add loaded carries into our basic work.

I name loaded carry workouts after birds in the raptor family. It started off as a joke about how we pick up the kettlebells and move them, but we soon found that this was a nice way of organizing them. The first workout is called the Sparrow Hawk or Sparhawk.

You will be doing goblet squats and suitcase carries. Suitcase carries are like farmer

Sparhawk Workout:

- 8 Goblet squats, then march away with the kettlebell in the left hand for about 60 feet (gym length is best).
- 7 Goblet squats, then march back to the original position with the kettlebell in the right hand.
- 6 Goblet squats, left hand suitcase walk.
- 5 Goblet squats, right hand walk.
- 4 Goblet squats, left hand walk.
- 3 Goblet squats, right hand walk.
- 2 Goblet squats, left hand walk.
- 1 Goblet squat, finished.

The workout has a total of 36 squats, but you are under load for about three minutes. Your anti-rotation muscles will be working overtime with the asymmetrical walking, and then they will still have to join in to support the squats. You will get the benefits of squatting including the mobility and flexibility work plus the additional boon of three minutes of time under tension.

Next, consider the "Cook Drill" from Gray Cook, P.T., founder of the Functional Movement System.

Stand while holding a kettlebell in the rack.

Now press the kettlebell straight overhead and walk. This is the waiter walk. Your arm should be completely straight, and your shoulder "packed" (pull it down, away from your ear).

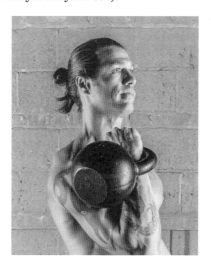
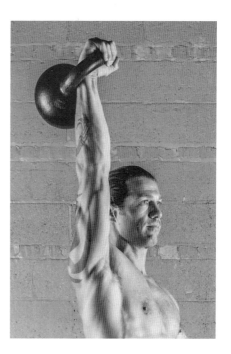

If you feel your arm start to wobble or your core start the shift, you've lost integrity. When that happens, bring the weight back to the rack position. Hold this position and continue to walk until you feel yourself losing integrity again. Then, release the weight to your side so that you're holding it like a suitcase. Once you can't hold the weight in that position, switch hands and start from the beginning of the drill (kettlebell overhead).

Gray recommends practicing this for up to 15 minutes, but we can also get plenty of a challenge by just going about 400 meters. What am I saying? We did that ONCE. Usually, we don't go very long, but occasionally this is a great drill all by itself.

Want more? Try the "CookED Drill". It is the same thing, but with added swings:

- Left hand waiter walk until nearing loss of integrity
- 10 Swings
- Left hand rack walk until nearing loss of integrity
- 10 Swings
- Left hand suitcase carry until nearing loss of integrity.
- 10 Swings

Repeat with the right hand.

One round has only sixty swings!!!

And sure, you can do it again or try it three times if you wish!

But, sometimes—like during the 10,000 Swing Challenge—you might want to circle a month and complete a challenge. Most of the time, you will want to do something like this daily:

1. Naked (unweighted) get-ups for five minutes.
2. Mobility sequence.
3. Practice few hip hinge drills and a few additional goblet squat prying movements.
4. Pick a single kettlebell workout from above. Time it, if appropriate.
5. Get-ups, one to five per side.
6. Sparhawk, Cook Drill or CookED Drill as a finisher.
7. Come back tomorrow!

THE FIRST TWENTY DAYS

> **Note:** A few years ago, I was asked to help someone transition from the HKC weekend to adding the HKC Three into their normal training. I offered the following as a guide for the next month or so after their HKC weekend. The person who requested the guide was concerned about passing an upcoming RKC because of the press standard, so note the addition of a fair amount of press practice. Certainly, push-ups could be used instead.

Fresh from a new learning experience, there is always a tendency to want to do everything all at once. That is tough to do and fraught with long and short-term issues. The first twenty days after the HKC experience is a chance to strive to master the movements and train the positions. Don't add speed and volume to poor movements: take your time to practice.

Prepping for the HKC is not as complex or as deep as the three-day RKC. Showing up "in shape" and ready to learn would be the best prep for the HKC, but I would include some additional mobility work and perhaps some work on the hinge, squat and basic rolling to prep for the event.

The time you spend prepping for the event pales in comparison to what you will do AFTER the HKC. The following twenty-day program can guide our HKC attendees deeper along the RKC path.

One note: during the HKC, I always include waiter walks and rack walks as part of the get-up section. From there, I demonstrate the one-arm press and introduce the kettlebell clean. This way, the participant has the tools for prepping the RKC. I trained for the RKC with the clean and press, swings and (what I thought were) snatches. So, I ask people to practice the press as soon as they can with kettlebells.

These twenty workouts can be done five days a week for a total of four weeks, or three days a week which sneaking up on two months. They can also be scheduled any way you choose. These workouts will provide the grounding for a solid base. Strive for mastery.

Daily Warm Up

It is generally a good idea to go through some mobility drills especially for these areas:

- Neck
- Shoulders
- Thoracic mobility
- Hips

Each week, take one day to do a full "toes to top" mobility workout.

It is recommended that you do the hip flexor stretch during each warm up and cool down period; it can be done very well along with an easy set of goblet squats. Many people find that a few easy sets of swings, a few goblet squats and a weightless set of one to five get-ups (on both sides) to be enough warm up.

Day One

- 3 Get-ups right side, 3 get-ups left side

- Practice the hip hinge
- Goblet squats: 2-3-5-2-3-5-2-3-5

Do Three Rounds:
- 15 Two-hand swings
- 1 Goblet squat
- 10 Reps high knee "march in place" (each time the right foot hits counts as one rep)
- Recovery breathing (up to 2 minutes)

- Five Minutes of Pressing Practice.

Day Two

- 2 Get-ups right, 2 get-ups left
- One arm press practice (Start with the "less strong arm" and alternate arms. One rep a rep with each hand) 1-2-3-1-2-3-1-2-3-1-2-3

Day Three

- 1 get-up right, 1 get-up left

Twenty minutes total:
- 30 Seconds of two-hand swings
- 30 Seconds of "Fast-Loose" drills

- Practice goblet squat

Day Four

- 10 Minutes of get-ups (alternate right and left sides)

Do Three Rounds:
- 15 Two hand swings
- 1 Goblet squat
- 10 Reps high knee "march in place" (each time the right foot hits counts as one rep)
- Recovery breathing (up to two minutes)

Day Five

- 5 Get-ups right, 5 get-ups left
- One arm press (start with "less strong arm" and alternate arms. One rep is a rep with each hand) 1-2-3-1-2-3-1-2

Day Six

- 3 Minutes of get-ups (alternate right and left sides)

Ten minutes total:
- 30 Seconds two hand swings
- 30 Seconds "Fast-Loose" drills

- Several sets of 5 goblet squats with a pause at the bottom

Day Seven

- 1 Get-up right, 1 get-up left

- One hand press practice (start with the "less strong arm" and alternate arms. "One rep" is a rep with each hand) 2-3-5-2-3-5-2-3-5

Day Eight

- Ten minutes of get-ups
- Practice the hip hinge
- Practice the goblet squat
- Practice the press

Day Nine

Do Five Rounds:
- 15 Two hand swings
- 1 Goblet squat
- 10 Reps high knee "march in place" (each time the right foot hits counts as one rep)
- Recovery breathing (for up to two minutes)

- One hand press practice (start with the "less strong arm" and alternate arms. "One rep" is a rep with each hand) 1-2-3-1-2-3-1-2

Day Ten

- 5 Get-ups right, 5 get-ups left

Five Minutes Total:
- 30 Seconds of two hand swings
- 30 Seconds "Fast-Loose" drills

- Goblet squats: 2-3-5-2-3-5

Day Eleven

- 5 Minutes of get-ups (alternate right and left sides)

- One hand press practice (start with the "less strong arm" and alternate arms. "One rep" is a rep with each hand) 1-2-3-5-1-2-3-5-3

Ten Minutes Total:
- 15 Seconds two arm swings
- 15 Seconds "Fast Loose" drills

DAY TWELVE
- 1 Get-up right, 1 get-up left

Five Minutes Total:
- 30 Seconds of two hand swings
- 30 Seconds "Fast-Loose" drills

- Goblet squats: 1-2-3-1-2-3-1-2

- One hand press practice (start with the "less strong arm" and alternate arms. "One rep" is a rep with each hand.) 1-2-3-1-2-3-1-2

DAY THIRTEEN
- 10 Minutes of get-ups (alternate right and left)

Do For Ten Rounds:
- 15 Two hand swings
- 1 Goblet squat
- 10 Reps high knee "march in place" (each time the right foot hits counts as "one rep")
- Recovery breathing (for up to two minutes)

DAY FOURTEEN
- 1 Get-up right, 1 get-up left

- One hand press practice (Start with "less strong arm" and alternate arms. "One rep" is one rep with each hand.) 2-3-5-2-3-5-2-3-5

DAY FIFTEEN
- 1 Get Up Right 1 Get Up Left

Five Minutes Total:
- 30 Seconds of two hand swings
- 30 Seconds "Fast-Loose" drills

- Goblet squats: 1-2-3-1-2-3-1-2

- One hand press practice (Start with "less strong arm" and alternate arms. "One rep" is one rep with each hand.) 1-2-3-1-2-3-1-2

Day Sixteen

Do Ten Rounds:
- 15 Two hand swings
- 5 Goblet squats
- 1 Push-up
- 10 Reps of high knee "march in place" (Each time the right foot hits counts as "one rep")
- Recovery breathing (for up to two minutes)

Day Seventeen

- 5 Minutes of get-ups (alternate right and left)

- One hand press practice (Start with "less strong arm" and alternate arms. "One rep" is one rep with each hand) 2-3-5-2-3-5-2-3-5

Day Eighteen

- 3 Get-ups right, 3 get-ups left

Twenty Minutes Total:
- 30 Seconds of two hand swings
- 30 Seconds "Fast-Loose" drills

Day Nineteen

- Goblet squats: 5-10-5-10-5

- One hand press practice (Start with "less strong arm" and alternate arms. "One rep" is one rep with each hand) 2-3-5-2-3-5-2-3-5

Day Twenty
- 1 Get-up right, 1 get-up left

Five minutes total:
- 30 Seconds of two hand swings
- 30 Seconds "Fast-Loose" drills

- Goblet squats: 1-2-3-1-2-3-1-2

- One hand press practice (Start with "less strong arm" and alternate arms. "One rep" is one rep with each hand) 1-2-3-1-2-3-1-2

So, there you go! The HKC is more than just the entry into the kettlebell world. It is the foundation of everything you will learn and the movements are the core to conditioning, mobility and goal achievement.

Welcome aboard.

Michael Warren Brown on the Program Minimum

In **Enter the Kettlebell,** a foundational protocol called the RKC Program Minimum is introduced. The program was developed by boxing coach Steve Baccari. His fighters needed a simple but effective routine that would not interfere with rigorous sports training.

The original program consists of a brief 10-minute warm-up of face-the-wall squats, pumps, and halos. Following the warm-up, the fighter did either a swing or get-up workout. Twice a week, they alternate swings with easy jogging, jump rope, or "Fast and Loose" drills for 12 minutes. Twice a week, the athletes do get-up singles, alternating sides every rep, for 5 minutes. Over time, feel free to increase the swing and get-up session times past 5 and 12 minutes.

The swing has been called the center of the kettlebell universe. All other ballistic lifts build from the swing. A clean is a swing that ends in the rack position. A snatch is a swing that is projected upward to an overhead lockout. The hike pass position of all ballistics looks identical, and all ballistics conclude with a violent hip snap and a full body plank. The only difference is the intention; with a swing, you think of throwing the kettlebell forward, but

The get-up is a full body lift that challenges many movement patterns: rolling, half kneeling, lunging—shoulder mobility and stability is simultaneously developed and challenged through many different angles. The shoulders must be properly prepared for the high volume pressing and snatching that comes with progressing through the RKC system.

There are countless ways to mix swings and get-ups into a program. The original "Program Minimum" is time tested and nearly fool-proof. Anyone will benefit from giving it a shot from time to time, regardless of their goals.

The original "Program Minimum" did not include goblet squats. Now, the one-day Hardstyle Kettlebell Certification is made up of the foundation of the entire RKC system: swings, get-ups, and goblet squats. These three moves performed with excellent technique and sharp focus will cover the majority of your client's goals.

At our gym, we always start with these three lifts along with several teaching drills for each. Once our athletes have mastered the fundamentals—and this process may take months or longer—we will introduce the clean and press, the snatch, and the double kettlebell front squat. The press builds on the foundation of the get-up. The clean and snatch build from the swing.

Keep in mind that the swing, get-up, and goblet squat are the true fundamentals. The best at any given skill are masters of the fundamentals. This means that the basics should take up the bulk of your training time. A common mistake people make is to rush into learning snatches and presses without giving the fundamentals their due.

We often revisit the original "Program Minimum" long after our athletes have become proficient in the fundamentals. I love to include two weeks of the "Program Minimum" after completing a challenging training block. The swings and get-ups seem to reward and heal the body after it has been heavily stressed. One of my favorite patterns is to run 1-2 weeks of "Program Minimum" followed by 6-8 weeks of hard hypertrophy training—followed by 1-2 weeks more of "Program Minimum." The lower volume and intensity of the "Program Minimum" allows for the body to compensate and recuperate.

All solid programs will include some waving of training variables (intensity, volume, or density). One classic variation is three hard training weeks followed by a deload week. For our more experienced athletes, we will often use a week of the "Program Minimum" as a deload.

So far, I have been discussing how we use the "Program Minimum" as it was initially written. Over time we have come up other ways to incorporate the principles of the program into training.

I am very slow to add anything to programs that are as simple and effective as the "Program Minimum." But, I think a few things can be introduced down the road to help keep the wheels of progress turning.

Here is a simple group of exercises: goblet squat, swing, get-up (and its drills), push-ups, and loaded carries. There are countless ways to incorporate these into a program but I'll give a few examples.

For the first example, I'll highlight two of Dan John's favorite principles:

> **If it is important, do it every day.**
>
> **The warm-up is the workout.**

I'll say it again, the swing, get-up, and the goblet squat are the foundation of the entire RKC system. They are so important that you will do them every single time you train. Now, the second part comes into play: the warm-up is the workout. You will touch all the moves in the warm-up every day, and then you will emphasize a single move as a short practice session.

An example warm-up incorporating the swing, get-up and goblet squat:
(The get-up is represented by our teaching drills. These are done with no kettlebell.)

- 10 Swings, 2 goblet squats, march in place
- Rolling 45's
- 10 Swings, 3 goblet squats, march in place
- Rolling T's
- 10 Swings, 5 goblet squats, march in place
- 5x From floor to kneeling windmill (left side)
- 10 Swings, 2 goblet squats, march in place
- 5x From floor to kneeling windmill (right side)
- 10 Swings, 3 goblet squats, march in place
- 5x Kneeling windmill to standing (left side)
- 10 Swings, 5 goblet squats, march in place
- 5x Kneeling windmill to standing (right side)
- 10 Swings, 2 goblet squats, march in place
- 1 Full get-up (left side)
- 10 Swings, 3 goblet squats, march in place
- 1 Full get-up (right side)
- 10 Swings, 5 goblet squats, march in place

(The squat progression is 2-3-5, 2-3-5, 2-3)

This sequence gives you 90 swings, 30 squats, and a lot of pattern work for the get-up. You can follow this portion with a short workout emphasizing one of the other lifts. You could easily include carries by simply doing a long "down and back" walk while working through the suitcase carries and waiter walks.

The Dan Martin "Program Minimum" is another example. Dan Martin first met Dan John at the famous Coyote Point Kettlebell Club. A retired firefighter and multi-sport athlete, Dan Martin tells us:

> "I was never much for warming up, but, I'm all for making my workouts more productive. Get-ups are my first exercise. Not doing them naked (without weight), but not doing them heavy either. Holding an 8-pound shot makes me concentrate.
>
> Then it's the DMPM (Dan Martin Program Minimum). Goblet squats x 5, push-ups x 5, two-hand swings x 15, Ring rows x 5. Suitcase walks for my finisher. Nothing fancy to be sure, but it's good enough, and good enough is like Manna from Heaven to me.
>
> I go walking on my "off" days. Afterwards I do the McGill Big 3 (curl up/bird dog/side plank).
>
> Just a few insights:
>
> Keeping it simple is key. There is no reason for me to do a lot of other exercises when all the bases are covered by the DMPM. I'm not all hung up on trying to fit my training into a seven-day week. Training can go every other day between lifting and walking or it may it will be two or three days in a row, and an off day here and there. Being able to train consistently is a privilege and I'm grateful."

Being able to consistently train is the brilliance of the "Program Minimum". Dan Martin is right to remind us that training is a privilege and we need to be grateful.

WHY CERTIFY?

As I review my half-century in the weight room (I started lifting in 1965), I begin to see our world of strength through the lens of something Arthur Schopenhauer noted:

> "When you look back on your life, it looks as though it were a plot, but when you are into it, it's a mess: just one surprise after another. Then, later, you see it was perfect."

With my massive collection of *Strength and Health* magazines and the short-lived *American Athlete* magazine, I can pick up an issue from just after World War II and see articles about how to repair the wounded warriors. The training presented for injured veterans is just like today's conventional training: laying down on machines, isolation work and a few sets of about eight to ten reps. While that kind of training is perfect for someone with compromised health and fitness, it's not optimal for elite sports performance!

I can read articles from the 1950s and see kettlebells used for leverage work, curls and grip training. I have found swing articles from the 1960s that emphasize a dangerous overflexion at the hinge and overextension at the plank.

Yes, kettlebell work had basically devolved into a mess. Powerlifting pushed Olympic lifting out of the way, and the bench press became the answer to every question. It wasn't a good answer. Some excellent coaches and trainers were pushing the strength envelope, but others were bogging us down. Speaking of bogging us down in the mess, one famous strength coach advocated using mud as resistance and noted "progress will be made." It works for pigs, so why not?

"Whadduya bench?" became the fitness standard. We saw the rise of the machines for leg training—as if leg presses indicated anything in the field of play or nature. The world of lifting was a mess.

And then, the kettlebell returned and all the credit—all the credit—goes to Dragon Door if you wish to be historically sincere. As an Olympic lifter, I couldn't fathom how these kettlebells could help me. I was surprised when I learned that the swing (done correctly and not how I first did it) made me a better Olympic lifter when I better understood the hinge. As much as I knew how to coach the squat, the horns on the kettlebell allowed me to teach how to push out the knees with the elbows. And then, I invented the goblet squat.

One arm pressing trumped most of the overhead work I was doing with throwers, since it demanded the hard work of the whole chain of anti-rotation muscles.

I became a better coach with kettlebells. But, I wouldn't have been ready for them when I first saw them in *Strength and Health*.

As if kettlebells were a part of my coaching life's plot, they arrived exactly when they needed to arrive...like what Gandalf says about wizards.

I learned enough to fill my head at my RKC certification in San Jose in 2008. Oddly, I learned even more a few months later as an assistant at an RKC at UCLA. And, I learned more again and again and again...

I started coaching in 1979, and thirty years later my head was being filled again!

I tell people all the time, you can't think through a ballistic movement. To understand the swing, snatch and clean, you need to "hear" the standards, drills, corrections, and the insights several times before it "clicks." Oddly, your technique might be seamless, but you might not be able to coach someone who has a simple error in their technique. Or, you might be able to "see" the problem, but your own technique is muddled.

When it comes to the goblet squat, get-up and press, are you really prying, packing or patterning the correct path? Or, are you just getting the reps in? Are you putting the kettlebell down like a professional every single time? How is your breathing? Your tension?

You need other eyes. You need community.

You need to recertify!

I work with a handful of RKCs daily. It is a rare few weeks when someone does NOT take me aside and point out a basic error that I'm making. On paper, I am a Master RKC—but in my own training, I am just another person swinging a kettlebell. I try not to get lazy. I try to stay packed and attack the hinge.

...But sometimes I don't.

Over time, skills degrade. "Safety is part of performance," except when we get tired, lazy or pressed for time. There are no excuses for lack of safety!

Getting certified, or recertified, will get eyes on you again. Recertifying for $500, for example, means three days of expert teaching and evaluation from at least three people, if not many, many more. This is a bargain compared to hiring a personal trainer.

Whenever anyone returns from a retreat, a clinic, conference, or workshop, the enthusiasm and excitement drips off of them. They have clear eyes and a missionary zeal.

When I first embarked on my RKC journey, I came home and converted everyone I knew to the "Kettlebell Crusade".

But, like all things, this wanes over time. It's not bad or good, but without community, without an ongoing dialogue, the battery runs out of excitement.

Outside of an annual visit to "Kettlebell Kamp", the best thing I can recommend is going to a certification.

For as much as I learn during the day, I think I learn more at night. At dinner, we exchange emails, gym insights, training mistakes, and fixes. A wealth of information seems to fit perfectly on a napkin. My favorite RKC dinner moments are when John Du Cane gives me a "MUST read" book recommendation. I am forever grateful for his recommendations.

John Du Cane does an interesting thing, when he asks for my book recommendations, he opens his phone and buys the books as I list them. If you believe in Shark Habits ("One bite!") like I do, then this is a good example to follow.

It's a rare day when I do NOT get a text, email, post, or message from someone I met at an RKC. It's nice to recommit to the shared experience. But, people still move on, drop off and walk away. Recertify your way into a new group of people who can walk the walk with you.

For example, if you were certified before 2008, you missed the goblet squat. Since then, the get-up has been revamped several times. Finally, I think we're teaching it with the appropriate steps, corrections, and drills. The sections on programming are tighter and clearer with more actual programs.

There are more swing drills and clearer correctives. In other words, the RKC is evolving. There was nothing wrong with the Sig Klein articles in *Strength and Health*, but kettlebells and kettlebell training has evolved. I rarely wear leopard skin and lace up boots when I train. (Note: I said when I train. My gym is judgment free, so you would be welcome to do what you need to do.)

I enjoy being part of this evolution. As much as I loved the original notion of the "kettlebell revolution," the kettlebell won. If you are keeping score, I enjoy the kettlebell evolution even more. Hundreds of people teaching thousands of clients with millions of swings will produce new insights, new ways of teaching and greater clarity with problems and issues.

I believe in investing in my continuing education. I sit in the front row at workshops and sign up for a weekend certification or conference at least once a year. It's hard to find a better deal than the $500 for the three-day RKC recertification.

In 1993, with two little girls in the house, I flew out for a week-long discus camp at Dennison University. For that week, Tiffini worked full-time along with fulfilling full-time mommy and daddy work. It cost a lot—money we didn't have—and it was a ton of work for me.

But, it changed my life. I have gone back every year since. It sharpened my coaching toolkit, opened my mind to new possibilities, and honed my own techniques.

In every way, we have earned back that investment.

Look at certification with the same lens. You will have a chance to fill your quiver of arrows, add new tools to your toolkit, experience a dynamic new community, learn new and evolving information, and get new sets of eyes on your technique.

The question shouldn't be "why certify?" it should be "why not?"

It is the perfect way to plot your career.

From the RKC manual:

There are four compelling reasons to recertify and keep your RKC status.

The number one reason to recertify is to keep your skill level up to the current standards of the RKC. This signifies the importance you place on continuing your education and keeping your personal athletic skills sharp.

The second reason to recertify is the obvious benefit you receive from the Dragon Door marketing machine by being listed as an RKC on the DragonDoor.com website. This can lead potential clients to you and give you a presence within and outside your own community.

The third reason to recertify is the ability to network with like-minded trainers. This is an extremely valuable tool to help keep you current, offer support and advice in all manners of kettlebell training and professional issues.

The fourth reason is to continue to receive a discount on kettlebell and Dragon Door kettlebell products. Orders can be placed by logging into your instructor account on DragonDoor.com where qualifying products are automatically discounted, or by calling Dragon Door Publications customer service at **1-800-899-5111** or internationally **214-258-0134**. You will be required to identify yourself as a currently certified instructor so that the phone agents will know to use your account to place your order.

About The Author

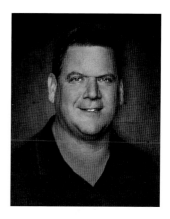

Dan John has spent his life with one foot in the world of lifting and throwing, and the other foot in academia. An All-American discus thrower, Dan has also competed at the highest levels of Olympic lifting, Highland Games and the Weight Pentathlon, an event in which he holds the American record..

Dan spends his work life blending weekly workshops and lectures with full-time writing, and is also an online religious studies instructor for Columbia College of Missouri. As a Fulbright Scholar, he toured the Middle East exploring the foundations of religious education systems. Dan is also a Senior Lecturer for St Mary's University, Twickenham, London.

His books, on weightlifting, include *Intervention*, *Never Let Go*, *Mass Made Simple* and *Easy Strength*, written with Pavel Tsatsouline as well as *From Dad, To Grad*. He and Josh Hillis co-authored *Fat Loss Happens on Monday*.

In 2015, Dan wrote *Can You Go?* on his approach to assessments and basic training. In addition, *Before We Go*, another compilation akin to Never Let Go became an Amazon Bestseller. In early 2017, Dan's book, *Now What?*, on his approach to Performance and dealing with "life," became a Bestseller on Amazon.

WHY THE Bodyweight Master™
FREE STANDING PULL UP BAR
is the ultimate solution for your upper body build out

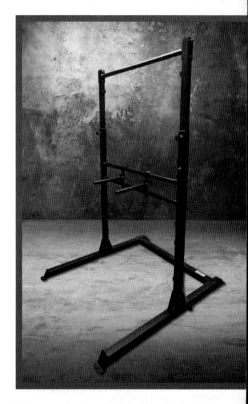

The noble Pull Up and the mighty Muscle Up are two bodyweight aristocrats that DO need a sturdy, indestructible piece of equipment to properly deliver their full, strength-enhancing benefits. Because to heap righteous slabs of etched meat on to your upper body—and get the military-industrial results you crave from your Pulls—you need the heavy-duty hardware to match your efforts…

But in the past, if you wanted to entertain bodyweight exercise royalty at home—and achieve the highest levels of Pull Up mastery—you would have been plain out of luck when it comes to a truly rugged, versatile and reliable free standing unit. Until now…

Enter the peerless *Bodyweight Master™ Free Standing Pull Up Bar,* designed by Dragon Door's calisthenics experts to specifically address the demands of the most hardcore bodyweight exercise fanatics. This unit looks tough and is tough—it reflects the inner and outer toughness of the user it is meant to serve…

We engineered our *Bodyweight Master™ Free Standing Pull Up Bar* to be the all-terrain, all-purpose battle tank of home exercise equipment… This thing does not take No for an answer—when it comes to rigorous abuse and a relentless quest for physical perfection…

And the *Bodyweight Master™* doubles up on your Dips, with detachable units and bars that allow all kinds of heights and challenges. Plus, at the top position, the Dip units let you set up for the more joint friendly neutral-grip Pull Up…

This is one investment in your health and strength that you can truly bank on—offering you year-upon-year of phenomenal physical gains and overall athletic enhancement!

Want to do low-bar work like Australian Pull Ups? Again, the *Bodyweight Master™* offers the perfect solution with its multiple low settings…

So: no more half-assed nonsense with jiggly rigs and ergonomically wretched devices that at best frustrate with weak, sub-par, inadequate results—and are usually doomed to become expensive coat hangers…

And no more door-frame wrecking, cheapo bars that limit your range of motion and cripple your athletic potential…

ADDITIONAL PRODUCT DETAILS:

- 2 detachable Dip units and bars which can be mounted at 7 different heights
- 1.5" diameter, 5" circumference Pull Up Bar
- 7 adjustable Pull Up bar heights: from 5' 2" to 8' 4"
- Easy assembly & disassembly
- 3' 11" wide x 4' 11.5" long base provides strong stability
- Wobble free
- Holes in the base allow unit to be screwed into the floor, for additional stability

Order Bodyweight Master™ online:
www.dragondoor.com/dbm001/

1•800•899•5111
www.dragondoor.com

24 HOURS A DAY
ORDER NOW

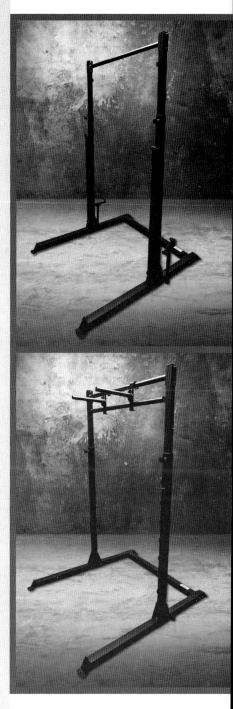

✓ RATED 10/10
...st what I was looking for
...Tom Gally / Yokohama, Kanagawa-ken, Japan

...had been trying for some time to find a freestand-... apparatus for pull-ups and dips that I could install ...y home. I had been thinking of getting a power ...k, but the ones available in Japan where I live ...e expensive and not quite what I needed. (I don't ...weights.)

...As soon as I saw this Bodyweight Master Free ...nding Pull Up Bar in a video by Al Kavadlo, I ...mediately ordered one (even though the shipping ...apan was more than the cost of the device!). It ar-... a week later, and it is exactly what I wanted. The ...embly instructions were clear and the assembly ...t smoothly.

...look forward to using it in my workout every day. ... apparatus is more solid and stable than I had ...ected, and it works well with pull-ups, dips, and ...raises. I was able to adjust the crossbar to a height ...t is just perfect for my own height and the height ...e ceiling.

...As noted in the description, it cannot be used with ...pension devices, swinging, or other moves that cre-... a lot of lateral momentum, as the device itself will ...e across the floor. (I haven't bolted it to the floor, ... I probably won't.)

✓ RATED 10/10
...odyweight Master Free Stand-
...g Pullup Bar
...Patrick Brunetti / Princeton, NJ

...Truly a great piece of equipment. Versatile and the ...st solid free standing bar I've found. You can do ...ypes of pullups, muscle ups, and the great human ... Set for multiple heights it's easy to use. Love the ...set up also.

...f you're looking for a complete piece of bodyweight ...ipment this is it.

✓ RATED 10/10
...xceeded my expectations!!
...Bob Abraham / San Diego, CA

...The Bodyweight Master Pull-Up Bar is a fantastic ...ition to any gym, home or otherwise. Solid, solid ...struction - ready for years of use and abuse. The ...ghened bar surface helps you get a good grip for ...w extra reps. And, icing on the cake - you can ...ckly change the pull-up bar to a dip station. Nothing ...positives to state about this piece of equipment.

✓ RATED 10/10
...mazing!!
...David Fumero / LA, CA, USA

...Combined with kettlebells, complete home gym!

✓ RATED 10/10
The best pull up bar on the market
By Shari Wagner / Denver, CO

I have wanted this pull up bar since I played with it at the Dragon Door Health and Strength Conference. It was so well made, and such a smart design. Its versatility is like nothing else out there on the market, and I had shopped around quite a bit. It's sturdy, yet doesn't take up a lot of room. It truly has it all.

✓ RATED 9/10
FANTASTIC purchase
By Dr. Alexander Ginzburg / Northbrook, IL

The item matches its description perfectly - and DragonDoor fully delivers. The versatility for positions of various pull-ups and dips is stunning, and does allow for most of Kavadlo brothers and Paul Wade's work now to BE attempted at home (or office).

✓ RATED 9/10
Great body weight exercise stand
By Zig Smith / Odenton, MD

Finally, an adjustable stand for dips and chin ups. The bench fit in a tight space very easily and it can be broken down easily. Great buy and it will last forever.

✓ RATED 9/10
Solid pull-up bar, perfect for kids
By Tim Henriques / Fairfax, VA

I ordered this as a Christmas present for my boys (7, 9, 10) who are really into exercising and working out, plus I wanted something for myself. It is solid and well-constructed. Here are some things I really like:

— Adjustable height, the lower height is great for kids
— The dip bars, you can make them any width you want and you can do pull-ups on them.
— When the pull-up bar is in the lowest position it is super stable
— It is great to hang a small punching bag (we have a 25 lb bag for them) from
— The bar itself has pretty good grip

I see this lasting a very long time

Bodyweight Master™ Free Standing Pull Up Bar

#dbm001 $399 plus $91

4 HOURS A DAY ORDER NOW   **1•800•899•5111**   **www.dragondoor.com**

▶ Order Bodyweight Master™ online: www.dragondoor.com/dbm001/

Add a Dragon Door Kettlebell to Your Arsenal—Durable, Resilient and Perfectly Designed to Give You Years of Explosive Gains in Strength, Endurance and Power

Even a man of average initial strength can immediately start using the 16kg/35lb kettlebell for two-handed swings and quickly gravitate to one-handed swings, followed by jerks, cleans and snatches. Within a few weeks you can expect to see spectacular gains in overall strength and conditioning—and for many—significant fat loss.

Dragon Door re-introduced kettlebells to the US with the uniquely designed 35lb cast iron kettlebell—and it has remained our most popular kettlebell. Why? Let Dragon Door's own satisfied customers tell the story:

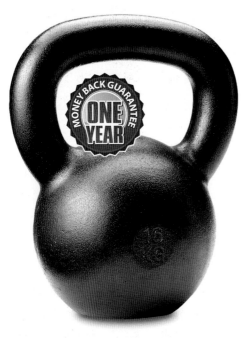

Our most popular kettlebell weighs 35lb (16kg)—and is the ideal size for most men to jumpstart their new cardio, conditioning and strength programs.

Excellent Quality

"Unlike other kettlebells I have used, Dragon Door is of far superior quality. You name it, Dragon Door has got it! Where other bells lack, Dragon Door kettlebells easily meet, if not exceed, what a bell is supposed to have in quality! Great balance, nice thick handle for grip strength, and a finish that won't destroy your hands when doing kettlebell exercises."
—BARRY ADAMSON, Frederick, MD

Continually Impressed

"Dragon Door never fails to impress with their quality service and products. I bought the 16kg last month and since adding it to my kettlebell 'arsenal', I am seeing huge improvement from the heavier weight. I have larger hands for a woman so the handle on the 16kg fits my hands perfectly and it feels great... This is my fifth month using kettlebells and I cannot imagine NOT using them. They have changed my life." —TRACY ANN Mangold, Combined Locks, WI

Dragon Door bells just feel better

"I purchased this 35lb bell for a friend, and as I was carrying it to him I was thinking of ways I could keep it for myself. Everything about this bell is superior to other brands. The finish is the perfect balance of smooth and rough. The handle is ample in both girth and width even for a 35 lb bell, and the shape/ dimensions make overhead work so much more comfortable. There is a clear and noticeable difference between Dragon Door bells and others. Now I am looking to replace my cheap bells with Dragon Door's. On a related note, my friend is thrilled with his bell."—RAPHAEL SYDNOR, Woodberry Forest, VA

Made for Heavy-Duty Use!

"These kettlebells are definitely made heavy-duty use! They are heftier than appear, and the centrifugal force gener while swinging single or two-handed requ correct form. I have read numerous or reviews of different companies who ma facture kettlebells, and it I have yet to a negative review of the kettlebells sold Dragon Door. I have both the 35 and 44 KBs, and I expect to receive a 53 lbs KB f Dragon Door by next week. And as I gai strength and proficiency, I will likely o the 72 lbs KB. If you like to be challer physically and enjoy pushing yourself, t buy a Russian Kettlebell and start swingi
—MIKE DAVIS, Newman, CA

New Dragon Door Bells Best Ever!

"Just received a new e-coat 16 yes day. Perfect balance, perfect textur non-slip paint, and absolutely seaml
—DANIEL FAZZARI, Carson City, NV

Dragon Door Kettlebells: T Real Deal!

"The differences between Dragon Do authentic Russian kettlebell and the infe one which I had purchased earlier at a l big box sports store are astounding! Dragon Door design and quality are cle superior, and your kettlebell just 'feels' r in my hand. There is absolutely no com ison (and yes, I returned the substanc hunk of iron to the big box store for a cr as soon as I received your kettlebell). I l forward to purchasing a heavier kettle from dragondoor.com as soon as I ma the 16kg weight!"—STEPHEN WILLIA Arlington, VA

Order Dragon Door Kettlebells online:
www.dragondoor.com/shop-by-department/kettlebells/

1•800•899•5111
www.dragondoor.com

24 HOURS A DA
ORDER NOW

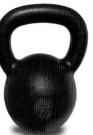

Are You Serious About Your Training?—Then Insist On Dragon Door's Premium RKC Kettlebells

Since 2001…Often Imitated, Never Equaled…

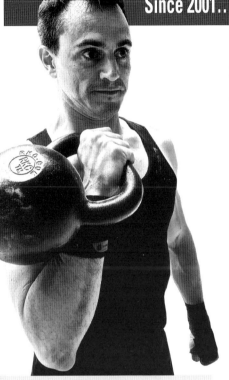

Size	Approx. Weight	Item #	Price
4 kg	(approx. 10 lbs.) Kettlebell	#P10N	$41.75 (plus s/h)
6 kg	(approx. 14 lbs.) Kettlebell	#P10P	$54.95 (plus s/h)
8 kg	(approx. 18 lbs.) Kettlebell	#P10M	$65.95 (plus s/h)
10 kg	(approx. 22 lbs.) Kettlebell	#P10T	$71.45 (plus s/h)
12 kg	(approx. 26 lbs.) Kettlebell	#P10G	$76.95 (plus s/h)
14 kg	(approx. 31 lbs.) Kettlebell	#P10U	$87.95 (plus s/h)
16 kg	(approx. 35 lbs.) Kettlebell Narrow Handle	#P10S	$96.95 (plus s/h)
16 kg	(approx. 35 lbs.) Kettlebell	#P10A	$96.75 (plus s/h)
18 kg	(approx. 40 lbs.) Kettlebell	#P10W	$102.75 (plus s/h)
20 kg	(approx. 44 lbs.) Kettlebell	#P10H	$107.75 (plus s/h)
22 kg	(approx. 48 lbs.) Kettlebell	#P10X	$112.75 (plus s/h)
24 kg	(approx. 53 lbs.) Kettlebell	#P10B	$118.75 (plus s/h)
26 kg	(approx. 57 lbs.) Kettlebell	#P10Y	$129.99 (plus s/h)
28 kg	(approx. 62 lbs.) Kettlebell	#P10J	$142.95 (plus s/h)
30 kg	(approx. 66 lbs.) Kettlebell	#P10Z	$149.99 (plus s/h)
32 kg	(approx. 70 lbs.) Kettlebell	#P10C	$153.95 (plus s/h)
36 kg	(approx. 79 lbs.) Kettlebell	#P10Q	$179.95 (plus s/h)
40 kg	(approx. 88 lbs.) Kettlebell	#P10F	$197.95 (plus s/h)
44 kg	(approx. 97 lbs.) Kettlebell	#P10R	$241.95 (plus s/h)
48 kg	(approx. 106 lbs.) Kettlebell	#P10L	$263.95 (plus s/h)
60 kg	(approx. 132 lbs.) Kettlebell	#P10I	$329.99 (plus s/h)

US ORDERING
- Kettlebells are shipped via UPS ground service, unless otherwise requested.
- Kettlebells ranging in size from 4kg To 24kg can be shipped to P.O. boxes or military addresses via the U.S. Postal Service, but we require physical addresses for UPS deliveries for all sizes 32kg and heavier.

Check on website or by phone for shipping charges.

ALASKA/HAWAII KETTLEBELL ORDERING
Dragon Door now ships to all 50 states, including Alaska and Hawaii, via UPS Ground. 32kg and above available for RUSH (2-day air) shipment only.

CANADIAN KETTLEBELL ORDERING
Dragon Door now accepts online, phone and mail orders for Kettlebells to Canada, using UPS Standard service. UPS Standard to Canada service is guaranteed, fully tracked ground delivery, available to every address in all of Canada's 10 provinces. Delivery time can vary between 3 to 10 business days.

24 HOURS A DAY ORDER NOW

1·800·899·5111
www.dragondoor.com

Order Dragon Door Kettlebells online:
www.dragondoor.com/shop-by-department/kettlebells/

Dragon Door's Premium, Heavy-Duty Kettlebell Rack is Built Like a Tank— Will Handle Your Complete Arsenal of Bells...

Convenience: Save space, keep it professional— with up to 1,400 lbs of kettlebells safely stored yet immediately available for your instant training needs...

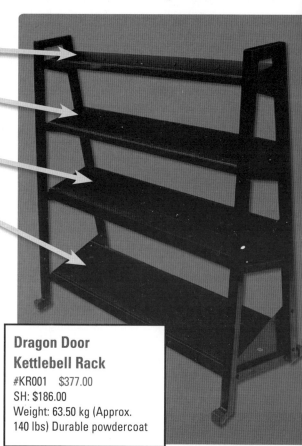

Top shelf can hold up to 80 kg (approx 176 lbs) of smaller kettlebells

Second shelf can hold up to 120 kg (approx 264 lbs) of medium-size kettlebells

Third shelf can hold up to 200 kg (approx 440 lbs) of medium/large-size kettlebells

Fourth shelf can hold up to 250 kg (approx 550 lbs) of large/extra large-size kettlebells

Enhanced safety feature: specially engineered to allow you to chain up your kettlebells—and avoid potential injury to young children or uneducated users.

Are you tired of kettlebells lying around all over your house or facility, taking up WAY too much space and messing with the professional elegance of your environment?

Would you like to have one simple, sturdy, safe yet highly accessible storage device for your kettlebells—that also LOOKS terrific?

As the proud possessor already of the world's premier kettlebells, don't you want to match them with the housing they deserve?

Then we invite to improve your training life with this magnificent Kettlebell Rack today…

Dragon Door Kettlebell Rack
#KR001 $377.00
SH: $186.00
Weight: 63.50 kg (Approx. 140 lbs) Durable powdercoat

ALMOST ¾ OF A TON OF LOAD-BEARING CAPACITY

Order Kettlebell Rack online:
www.dragondoor.com/kr001

1•800•899•5111
www.dragondoor.com

24 HOURS A DAY
ORDER NOW

Customer Acclaim for Dragon Door's Bestselling 12kg/26lb Kettlebell

Converted Gym Rat....

"I have seen DRASTIC changes EVERYWHERE on my body within a very short time. I have been working out religiously in the gym for the past 15 years. I have seen more change in JUST 1 month of kettlebell training. KB's build bridges to each muscle so your body flows together instead of having all of these great individual body parts. The WHOLE is GREAT, TIGHT and HARD. Just what every woman wants."
—Terri Campbell, Houston, TX

Best Kettlebells Available

"Okay, they cost a lot and, with the shipping costs, it's up there. However, the local kettlebells were far inferior in quality—do you want rough handles when you're swinging? And, if you order a cheaper product online, you won't even KNOW the quality until you have them. Dragon Door kettlebells are well formed, well-balanced and have no rough edges. Sometimes you just have to go with the best and these are the best!"
—Judy Taylor/ Denver, CO

Awesome tool for the toolbox!!!

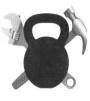

"I took some time off from grappling to focus on strength using my new kettlebells... Needless to say my training partners knew something was up. My 'real' total body strength had increased dramatically and I had lost about 5 pounds of bodyfat weight. We are getting more!!!!"
—Jason Cavanaugh, Marietta, PA

More Fun Than a Dumbbell or Barbell

"Very satisfied. A lot of fun. Indestructable. Delivered quickly. Much more fun to use than dumbbells or barbells. Everytime I see the bells I pick them up and do something with them. Great!"—Sonny Ritscher, Los Angeles, CA

Beautiful Cast Iron

"The casting was so well done that the kettlebell doesn't look like a piece of exercise equipment."—Robert Collins, Cambridge, MA

Changing a 64 year old's life!

"After being very fit all my life with everything from Tae Kwon Do to rock climbing and mountain biking, I hit 60 ... had a heart valve repair and got horribly out of condition, It was difficult for me just to get up off the floor when I sat to put wood in the wood burning fireplace. In just 6 weeks with a 12 kilo kettlebell I've improved dramatically. The 'real life' strength that you develop is amazing. The difference to your 'core' is dramatic. Wish I'd discovered kbells years ago!"—Lowell Kile, Betchworth, United Kingdom

I Love My Kettlebell!

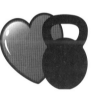

"I am really enjoying my kettlebell. When I received mine, I was so pleased with the finish and the handle. It is definitely a high quality product and when I work my strength up, I will order my next kettlebell from DragonDoor as well."—Diana Kerkis, Bentonville, AR

GREAT Piece of Equipment

"Excellent quality and finish. I'm a runner who doesn't do heavy weights; this 26 lb. KB is a great addition to my training and has made a meaningful difference, even in the first few weeks. Something about the shape INVITES you to work with it!

Highly recommended."—Matthew Cross, Stamford, CT

Maximum Results

"There is not a product around that compares to the 26 lb kettlebell. It is a health club, of its own. In my opinion anybody of any age or fitness level can achieve results. "—Jim Thoma, Shoreline, WA

The Handler

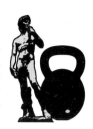

"The Kettlebell is the authority of weights. I'm 50 years old and have been working out since I was 12. I purchased the 12kg kettlebell, and at the present time used it for six different exercises. Its shape makes such a big difference; you can be creative using it to strengthen areas of your body simultaneously in one motion. In the future I will purchase the 35 kg."
—Ronald Bradley, Alpharetta, GA

Excellent Product

"I have bought two other (competitor's) kettlebells since the purchase of this product, and there's an obvious difference in quality. I am very pleased with the purchase from Dragondoor. Thanks."
—Steve Crocker, Coupeville, WA

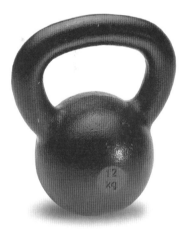

Russian Kettlebell - 12kg (26 lbs.)
Authentic Russian kettlebell, w/rust resistant e-coat #P10G $76.95

24 HOURS A DAY ORDER NOW
1•800•899•5111
www.dragondoor.com

Order Dragon Door Kettlebells online:
www.dragondoor.com/p10g